Praise for *True Wellness*

"Finally, a book examining Western and Eastern approaches to medicine in one text. This great book not only dispels the myth that a huge chasm exists between each medical model but explores the concept that they are more similar than anyone has ever been willing to examine or admit.

"The authors discuss the history of both the Western and Eastern practice of medicine. They then do something no one has ever done by documenting the convergence of the two.

"You will never see qi and cell biology discussed in the same text except here. It is a refreshing and eye-opening view. This isn't a text about choosing between Western and Eastern medicine but integrating both in complementary fashion.

"I teach evidence-based medicine and population health from the Western approach. I'm also a martial artist and author who writes about Eastern principles of thought. Seeing the fusion of these worlds is quite insightful, as it is done in academic fashion, filled with critical thought about the benefits of understanding the symbiosis of these models.

"The integration of Western and Eastern medical models the authors describe is groundbreaking. It should be a part of current medical education. People will be healthier, and medical practitioners will be wiser by reading this book."

—Dr. Phillip Stephens, author, *Emergency Medicine: The Inside Edge*

"The authors have done a great job explaining how people can benefit from utilizing Western and Eastern medicine together to create better health and wellness. It should be required reading for medical, osteopathy, ARNP, and PA students. The qigong movements are easy to follow and a wonderful introduction to Eastern exercise. I plan on incorporating these principles into my daily practice of medicine."

—Robert E. Ford, MD, specializes in family medicine (internal medicine, gynecology, pediatrics, orthopedics, emergency medicine) and personal injury

T0266319

"Beautifully written book. Full of valuable information for both medical professionals and the lay community. Easy step-by-step instruction on how to achieve your 'true wellness.' This book is sure to become a classic!"

—Gerald J. Leglue Jr., MD, FAAPMR, FAAMA, president,
American Academy of Medical Acupuncture

"*True Wellness* offers an essential paradigm shift in the world of health care, encouraging unity across disciplines for both physicians and patients who want to combine the best options for alleviating symptoms and addressing the root cause of disease. It suggests a fundamental accountability that every person must take for their well-being and gives a plan of action to begin. In the increasingly complex world of medicine, Kurosu and Kuhn's blending of science and humanism is a much-needed illustration of the potential for good when different vantage points work together toward a unified goal."

—Jennie Lee, author, *True Yoga: Practicing with the Yoga Sutras
for Happiness and Spiritual Fulfillment* and *Breathing Love:
Meditation in Action*

"Drs. Kurosu and Kuhn are uniquely qualified to blend the art and science of Eastern and Western medicine. They examine the benefits of both disciplines and make persuasive arguments to integrate these two great healing traditions. Thoughtfully presented and articulately written, *True Wellness* leads the reader to understand and develop skills that enhance their well-being—now and for a lifetime."

—Joseph M. Helms, MD; founding president, American Academy
of Medical Acupuncture; president, Helms Medical Institute;
author, *Acupuncture Energetics: A Clinical Approach for Physicians*
and *Getting to Know You: A Physician Explains How Acupuncture
Helps You Be the Best You*

"This book was written by two highly experienced practitioners of health and healing. It fulfills the promise to understandably combine Western and East Asian medicine. The text has just enough Western science to form a balance with the Daoist philosophy that underpins Chinese medicine. This enables the reader to understand how relatively simple steps can be effective in treating complex health situations. Few authors have taken such a wide-ranging approach that effectively addresses medical care, philosophy, history, and culture. I am impressed."

—Michael M. Zanoni, PhD, LAc,
diplomate in Oriental medicine (NCCAOM)

"*True Wellness* is a refreshing, well-informed, and well-presented discussion about a holistic approach to health that integrates both Eastern and Western methods. All too often, works of this type are exercises in hyperbole, breathless revelations of esoteric Eastern secrets, a Gospel or Prosperity for the Body that promises magical benefits for the true believer. What Drs. Kurosu and Kuhn present as a welcome antidote is a measured, sober, well-informed, and well-argued volume that provides a pathway toward integrating different approaches to health.

"Particularly for individuals involved with Eastern disciplines like the martial arts or yoga, the personal experience of the benefits of practice suggests that there is something to the mystical claims embedded in the philosophical treatises of the East. Qi or prana appears to be a force we experience fleetingly in our practice: real, yet elusive as smoke. How best to explain this?

"In *True Wellness*, the authors lay out a conceptual model that presents life and health as a dynamic process of energy management. Both Eastern and Western traditions acknowledge this as a fact, but they describe the processes in very different ways. In modern Western medicine, for example, the biomedical model stresses disease as something that is caused at the molecular level. Eastern approaches view the body as a microcosm of the universe, stressing the interconnectedness of various factors.

"The strength of this book is that the authors acknowledge the respective strengths (and weaknesses) of both systems. Western medicine is unparalleled in specific treatments for discrete health issues; Eastern approaches focus on the interrelationship of factors. As a result, Kurosu and Kuhn are candid in their discussion of what Eastern approaches can bring to the table. Acupuncture is a case in point. While there appear to be real benefits to the practice and some intriguing research about electrical conductivity at acupuncture points and possible physiological responses to stimulation, the authors are candid in noting that the meridians and energy channels posited by Eastern traditions remain elusive in terms of scientific standards. While they note associated effects from acupuncture, the specific physiological mechanism associated with these effects has not been completely discovered.

"As a result, the authors wisely advocate for the integration of both traditions in the promotion of health. Where real benefits can be obtained from Eastern approaches, they can and should be incorporated into medical treatment. Certainly, the awareness of the complex interplay between diet, lifestyle, exercise, and other factors is by now widely acknowledged in the West. Eastern approaches may well offer additional benefits to what is sometimes a clinical and overtly fragmented Western approach.

"In the end, the authors advocate a refreshingly grounded perspective: remain open to new possibilities; use common sense; engage in moderation, good habits, and balance. Their chapter on steps to optimal health provides a good framework for those looking to apply these insights, advocating a step-by-step approach to evaluation and action. The subsequent chapter on goal setting provides readers with a blueprint that can lead from reflection to action. Appendices on topics like diet and glycemic index and load are also useful.

"In short, *True Wellness* is a well-conceived, well-written guide to a holistic approach to health and wellness. It combines the well-informed and measured approach of scientifically trained clinicians with the insights and possibilities inherent in non-Western approaches to health. What is most refreshing is the clear and levelheaded approach they advocate. The approach should be familiar to any individual following the disciplines of the East: remain open to possibility; be aware, reflective, and willing to engage in the hard and important work involved with the pursuit."

—John Donohue, PhD, martial artist, author of numerous books
about martial arts as well as martial art fiction

CATHERINE KUROSU, MD, LAc
AIHAN KUHN, CMD, OBT

TRUE
WELLNESS

How to Combine the
Best of Western and Eastern Medicine
for Optimal Health

YMAA Publication Center
Wolfeboro, NH USA

YMAA Publication Center, Inc.
PO Box 480
Wolfeboro, New Hampshire 03894
1-800-669-8892 • info@ymaa.com • www.ymaa.com

ISBN: 9781594396304 (print) • ISBN: 9781594396311 (ebook)

Managing Editor: T. G. LaFredo
Cover design: Axie Breen
This book typeset in Minion Pro and Frutiger.

10   9   8   7   6   5   4   3   2   1

Publisher's Cataloging in Publication
Names: Kurosu, Catherine, author. | Kuhn, Aihan, author.
Title: True wellness : how to combine the best of Western and Eastern
    medicine for optimal health / Catherine Kurosu, Aihan Kuhn.
Description: Wolfeboro, NH USA : YMAA Publication Center, [2018] |
    Includes bibliographical references and index.
Identifiers: ISBN: 9781594396304 | 9781594396311 (ebook) |
    LCCN: 2018951323
Subjects: LCSH: Self-care, Health. | Alternative medicine. |
    Health behavior. | Well-being. | Nutrition. | Food preferences. |
    Vitamins. | Dietary supplements. | Medication abuse—Prevention. |
    Exercise. | Qigong. | Meditation. | Acupuncture. | Health—Alternative
    treatment. | Mind and body. | Holistic medicine. | Medicine, Chinese. |
    BISAC: HEALTH & FITNESS / Healthy Living. | HEALTH & FITNESS /
    Health Care Issues. | MEDICAL / Alternative & Complementary Medicine.
Classification: LCC: RA776.95 .K87 2018 | DDC: 613.2—dc23

NOTE TO READERS
The practices, treatments, and methods described in this book should not be used as an alternative to professional medical diagnosis or treatment. The authors and publisher of this book are NOT RESPONSIBLE in any manner whatsoever for any injury or negative effects that may occur through following the instructions and advice contained herein.

It is recommended that before beginning any treatment or exercise program, you consult your medical professional to determine whether you should undertake this course of practice.

Printed in Canada

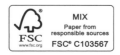

Contents

For my parents, Anna and Allen Bloom,
with gratitude for your unending support,
encouragement,
and love.
And for Rob and Hannah,
with appreciation for your infinite patience.

For my husband, Gerry Kuhn,
and my children, Sharon and Peter.

Foreword

I CANNOT THINK OF A TIMELIER TOPIC than True Wellness. I have been working in the "alternative medicine" field for the past thirty years and I have been frustrated with the health-care crisis we have in America. We have incredible technology and excellent doctors, but the system is geared toward acute care and sickness care. There is too much emphasis on treating symptoms and too little emphasis on helping patients learn how to get well and stay well. Sadly, there is more profit in keeping people sick. We need a better approach. Dr. Kurosu and Dr. Kuhn have both been trained in Eastern and Western medicine and they understand how to integrate the strengths of both disciplines. The authors make a strong argument for a new paradigm while offering an easy to understand guide for maintaining true wellness.

After laboring for years in traditional addictions treatment, I discovered intriguing research on using brain wave training to treat alcoholism. When I started implementing a brain-based approach in my treatment center, I experienced amazing transformations. This led me to embark on a career path of neurofeedback therapy, which is based on science and supported by professional literature, yet still regarded as experimental and non-reimbursable. Neuroscience has taught us about neuroplasticity and the brain's remarkable ability to rewire itself. Regardless of diagnosis, when the brain works better, everything works better. Conversely, when the body works better, the brain works better. Eastern medicine has known this for centuries. When I had an opportunity to work with a skillful acupuncture physician we both discovered that the ancient wisdom of oriental medicine was very compatible with the modern technology of training the brain. The two modalities have a synergistic effect. This was my first experience with "East meets West" in medicine and it inspired me to learn more.

Today we have the science and technology to verify and understand the validity of Eastern concepts of qi and traditional practices of mindful movement. For those of us raised in Western society it may not be easy to grasp the concept of subtle energies and non-invasive health practices. How do we reconcile the daily messages delivered by Big Pharma through the media, with the idea that there are valid non-pharmaceutical approaches to health care? The answer is in communication and education.

It wasn't until I went through my own health crisis that I was able to put it all together. Under the illusion of robust health and infallibility, a combination of unusual stress, inflammation, sleep apnea, and a tiny virus suddenly put me into a life-threatening heart condition. It took a combination of Eastern and Western medicine to restore me to health. I now understand how integrative medicine can work for anyone. This book presents an exquisite explanation of how to utilize and integrate the strengths of both approaches to achieve and maintain true wellness.

My clinical and personal experiences led me to develop an integrative wellness center with a team of talented practitioners who collectively can treat, educate, and guide clients into true wellness. As part of this journey, I invited Dr. Kuhn to bring qigong into our program. I found her to be an amazing teacher and healer. Her energy, grace, balance, and strength were a testament to the wellness life style she embraces. We have subsequently collaborated on natural healing conferences with an emphasis of combining Eastern and Western approaches. The message is well received, because people are frustrated with our sickness care system and are seeking a better way. Herein is a better way.

I urge everyone to read this book and embrace its message. It is more than a text. It is a workbook that can help the reader to take charge of personal well-being. Whether one is suffering from illness, curious, skeptical, or already on a path of wellness, there is something of value in the following chapters for any reader. It is through education and communication that we can make informed decisions and take charge of our health.

George Rozelle, PhD, QEEGD, BCN, Senior fellow
MindSpa Integrative Wellness Center
Sarasota, Florida

Foreword

"EVERYTHING OLD IS NEW AGAIN." This was the quote I was reminded of while reading through this exceptionally well-researched work on how the principles of Eastern and Western medicine can be combined to create a wellness regimen for everyone. As a physician, trained in Western medicine in the heyday of the scientific method, I have always been interested in why some of my patients chose "alternative therapies" and was often frustrated in my lack of knowledge to answer their questions. This book, while written for patients, provides all readers with a historical perspective on how the Eastern and Western medical traditions developed, and why they are not as opposed to each other, as some would presume based on their location on a navigational compass. As the medical system struggles to reinvent itself for the future, this look back is an opportunity to remind us all that we don't have to choose one system over the other. For instance, rather than refer to Eastern medicine as "alternative" some schools have moved to rename their departments as "integrative" medicine. When patients learn that their providers are being trained in a system that acknowledges the benefits of both Eastern and Western medicine, this will hopefully lead them to be more open in telling their physicians what therapies they have already tried. While my understanding of Eastern medicine has remained rudimentary over the years, I have seen the benefits that it has provided to my patients first hand, often performed by Dr. Kurosu herself!

This book will provide patients and physicians a common vocabulary and will empower patients to take control of their health. By emphasizing healthy eating and by including a series of homework exercises, it serves as a practical guide. The discussion of motivation to make changes is especially useful to encourage patients, in light of the non-linear method through which behavioral change occurs. *True Wellness* is a comprehensive guide for anyone who desires to improve their wellness, and that is a concept that physicians and patients both need. Given the modern crisis of physician burnout, the principles in this book are applicable to all. We need to rediscover the holistic concepts of the past in order to create a new model that combines the Eastern and Western traditions in an integrative fashion to improve health care for all.

Holly Olson, MD, MACM, FACOG, Deputy Designated
Institutional Official for Graduate Medical Education,
John A. Burns School of Medicine, Honolulu, Hawai'i

Preface

LIFE IS ABOUT ENERGY MANAGEMENT. Human existence may also include acts of kindness, heroism and compassion, artistic creation, and athletic achievement, but none of that can happen without adequate energy. Our existence revolves around procuring, preparing, and consuming food, moving through our day productively, then sleeping to allow our brains and body to repair and function efficiently the next morning. In short, we take in energy and then expend it. When the body can't take in sufficient energy or process it correctly, a shortfall results. If uncorrected, this lack of energy feeds a vicious cycle, dampening our metabolism, disrupting our sleep, and eventually leading to disease.

Whether you look at health and disease through the lens of Western or Eastern medicine, energy management is at the heart of the matter. A Western physician is concerned about the biochemistry of cellular metabolism as a function of energy utilization, whereas the Eastern practitioner is interested in the flow of energy throughout the channels and organ systems of the body.

It is our contention that all these healers are talking about the same phenomena.

Western and Eastern medical systems share a common foundation: the understanding that humans are energetic beings. What differs is the way in which these energetic processes are described. Millennia ago, practitioners of either paradigm had no access to biochemical tests, magnetic resonance imaging, or electrocardiograms. The light microscope wasn't even invented until a few hundred years ago. Each group, half a world apart, had to develop a logical system of medicine to care for their people; each system was based on the prevailing culture. As we shall see, each culture's worldview shaped its approach to health and healing. Our purpose in writing this book is to show that, as is often the case between competing factions, Western and Eastern medicine have more commonalities than differences.

Certainly, all practitioners strive to give the best care and attention to their patients, no matter the approach. The goal is to help patients live well through optimal energy management. This is just another way of describing how today both Eastern and Western health practitioners counsel patients to choose nutritious food, exercise regularly, practice qigong or tai chi, meditate daily, and sleep sufficiently. All these endeavors affect the quality and quantity of energy in the body and the manner in which it is expended. This is what allows a person to go beyond merely existing; to focus the mind and harness the creative spark that gives rise to a symphony, a ballet, or a painting; to care for our families with love and compassion; and to contribute our time and efforts to bettering society for all of its members.

Can blending Western and Eastern medicine do all that? We believe the answer is a resounding "Yes!" As physicians trained in both Western and Eastern healing systems, we understand how to use the strengths of each to meet the needs of the individual patient. Over the years, our patients have learned how to use Eastern methods to treat Western diseases and have achieved amazing results. By incorporating acupuncture, qigong, tai chi, and meditation into their standard care, our patients have optimized all aspects of their health.

We do not share a medical practice, but when we met in 2009, we immediately saw our similarities and the potential to collaborate. We are both Western-educated medical doctors. As it happens, we both specialized in gynecology and obstetrics, and also trained as practitioners of Eastern medicine. We saw how our patients had struggled within the national health-care system before adding Eastern methodologies into their daily routines. These people were suffering with all the chronic diseases that are rampant in America, such as diabetes, heart disease, chronic pain syndromes, and cancer. We saw our patients improve their quality of life and reduce their disease burden by taking control of their health and including Eastern practices.

But, we also saw the effort required. Some patients were absolute self-starters. All they needed was the right information and they sprang into action. These people were the exceptions. We knew that making fundamental lifestyle changes is difficult for most people, and they require continued guidance and encouragement along the way. With the complexity and expense of the current medical system, it is often not possible for Western health-care practitioners to give the patient this attention. Even with physician extenders, such as nurse practitioners or physician assistants, there is a shortage of medical providers in many areas of the country. As a consequence, there simply isn't enough time in an average medical appointment for these healers to effectively counsel and cajole a patient into making these huge shifts in self-care—but these huge shifts are exactly what are needed to turn the tide of chronic illness, individually and nationally.

This book, which is the first of a series, will help you lay the foundation for lasting health. Our hope is that you, the reader, will be inspired to take matters into your own hands. The general guidelines presented here can be applied universally. Startling improvements can be made in almost every chronic illness. For those who may still need specialized treatment plans for specific conditions, the upcoming series of books will offer unique insights, in-depth discussion, and a precise integrative approach for a variety of chronic ailments.

Books cannot substitute for a caring medical provider, but our intent with this initial installment is to help you take that first step toward wellness. Throughout these pages we offer our shared perspective on the nature of real well-being and offer some personal reflections based on the experiences of our patients.

Chapter by chapter, we walk you through this integrative approach to care, on your way to improved health. Through an understanding of the history and philosophy of Western and Eastern medicine, you will see the similarities. By examining some of the scientific evidence that explains energetic phenomena, you will recognize the factors in your daily life that can make an enormous impact on your well-being. In taking a short detour to comprehend the complexity of this country's medical system, you will find your role within it and learn how to navigate that industry more effectively. After learning more about the benefits and safety of Eastern medicine, you will be presented with strategies for speaking with your doctor and creating a therapeutic alliance within your own multidisciplinary health-care team.

Finally, in the last chapter, we provide tools to help you solve your health challenges. Step-by-step, using techniques derived from both Western and Eastern medicine, you will discover how to breathe, think, and act in ways that will be energetically transformative. You will be able to prepare and implement a healing plan that you can sustain. We are confident that the healthy choices you make each day will lead to a lifetime of optimal health for you, your family, and your community. We wish you true wellness.

Catherine Kurosu, MD, LAc
Aihan Kuhn, CMD, Dipl. OBT

CHAPTER 1

Medicine in Evolution

E VERY CIVILIZATION HAS SEARCHED for the cause of disease. In ancient times, throughout the world, it was thought that illness originated with the supernatural. A person who became sick was either possessed by an evil spirit or being punished by a god. Every society had its own myths, legends, and explanations regarding disease. The "doctor" of the tribe was a shaman, a spiritual leader who also had the ability to heal. By blending an understanding of human nature, community, and the physical world, shamans created rituals and potions that could cure all ills, or so they thought.

Gradually the role of the shaman was subdivided into two—the spiritual leader and the physical healer. Over time, and in different societies, these roles overlapped to varying degrees, but the realization that diseases were not caused by mystical events marked a significant conceptual shift. Doctors started to look at the natural world around them to explain why people became sick.

At the beginning of the formal history of medicine, whether Eastern or Western, the physician viewed the patient as a complete person. Rather than focusing on only the physical aspects of a patient's illness, the ancient physician was acutely aware of the emotional and spiritual dimensions of disease. Doctors recognized that having a medical condition could affect a person's emotional and spiritual state. Conversely, emotions and spirituality could influence the course of a given disease. Additionally, the physician knew that each patient was part of a family and a society that would certainly influence that person's state of health. It was also understood that the person's well-being had a great deal to do with their daily habits and how those habits affected their internal energy. It was the duty and privilege of the physician to assist their patients in achieving optimal health. That meant not simply recovering from illness but, more important, maintaining good health.

The following is a brief explanation of how Western biomedical philosophy and education has strayed from that path and how Eastern medicine has never faltered.

The History and Philosophy of Western Medicine

Today, Western medicine is considered to be the practice of medicine as performed in modernized, industrialized countries all across the globe. Other names for this sort of medicine are allopathy or biomedicine. This system generally favors the use of the latest technologies and tends to focus on the alleviation of symptoms. Western medicine can trace its lineage back to ancient Greece, but there the central idea of how to practice medicine was the opposite of the manner in which Western medicine is practiced today. Thousands of years ago, it was understood that to successfully treat a patient, one did not just relieve their symptoms. The underlying abnormality that started the disease process had to be discovered. Once this was found, the problem could be solved. In ancient Greece, and all other similar civilizations, physicians knew that treating the symptom would result in only temporary relief, but unearthing the root cause of a disease could lead to a lasting cure.

The father of Western medicine is considered to be Hippocrates, a Greek doctor who lived from 460 to 360 BCE. Hippocrates felt that in order to care for a patient, he had to understand the patient's way of life and particular constitution. He emphasized balance in daily living with respect to food, drink, and exercise. Disease was thought to be an imbalance of material substances within the human body, specifically blood, water, and bile. These substances were called "humors." These humors also were associated with qualities (hot, cold, moist, and dry) and elements (earth, air, fire, and water). Hippocrates considered "health" to be the perfect balance of the humors, qualities, and elements within each person.

Even before Hippocrates, Greek philosophers and physicians were very interested in the natural world and, like the Chinese, used observations of the natural world to explain human growth and development. Two such philosopher-physicians, Pythagoras and Alcmaeon (circa 500 BCE), felt that the universe was made up of pairs of opposite qualities, such as hot/cold and moist/dry. Harmony within these pairs was considered to be all-important, as an imbalance would result in disease. This is mirrored in the Chinese theory of yin and yang, which we discuss in greater detail shortly.

Another similarity between Eastern medical theory and early Western medical thought lies in the concept of "vitalism." This is the idea that there is within the human body an active and intelligent force that instinctively maintains and repairs the health of each person. This "vital force" could be considered equivalent to the Chinese concept of "qi." The tenets of vitalism can be seen within several disciplines of medicine that arose from Western medicine, such as homeopathy and chiropractic.

The idea of a dynamic energy within an individual began to lose favor in Europe after the Renaissance and during the Scientific Revolution (1450–1630 CE). Advancing technology gave physicians of this era the tools to examine ever more intricate workings of the human body, and more and more of its mysteries were solved. Increasing attention was paid to anatomic dissection and localized disease processes.

Prior to the invention of the light microscope in 1609 and the identification of bacteria, it was thought that diseases arose spontaneously without a discernible cause. This was called the theory of "spontaneous generation." Even though microorganisms could be seen under the light microscope, many believed that these creatures arose spontaneously. From the mid-1600s onward, some scientists tried to disprove this theory. Italian scientists Francesco Redi (1626–1697) and Lazzaro Spallanzani (1729–1799) performed experiments that discredited the theory of spontaneous generation, but there were still those who found fault with their experimental design. Finally, in 1858, it was the experiments of Louis Pasteur, a French professor of chemistry, that disproved the theory of spontaneous generation and then later demonstrated that infectious diseases were caused by microorganisms. With the work of Pasteur, a German scientist named Robert Koch, and other notable European investigators, modern germ theory was brought to fruition.

Because bacteria, viruses, and molds could cause infectious diseases, an understanding of these microbes eventually led to many treatments that could cure these illnesses. Vaccines were created to prevent contracting a disease in the first place.

The study of microbiology and the development of antibiotics and vaccines are some of the most important discoveries of Western medicine. Countless deaths have been avoided as a result. It is highly likely that each of us knows someone whose life has been saved by the use of antibiotics.

As undeniably remarkable as these discoveries were, it is interesting to note that, from the 1800s onward, the study of medicine changed. It became centered on the search for the simplest, single explanation for the cause of an illness. This is quite understandable, given that these discoveries were made in the midst of the Industrial Revolution in Europe. At this time, factories emerged, and each part of the production process was broken down and compartmentalized. No longer did an artisan see the creation of an item through from start to finish. Rather, a worker manufactured one portion of an item and passed it on to the next worker for completion.

This idea of fragmentation became pervasive in Western medicine. The ability to break down biochemical or physiologic processes into smaller and smaller components has led to an astonishingly deep understanding of the human body. This led to the rise of the physician-scientist. Historically, in America, many doctors were trained to use a more practical type of medicine that involved natural botanical remedies; the curriculum of a great number of medical schools in the United States at the end of the 1800s fell into this category. Unfortunately, some of these schools advertised to and accepted any student who could pay the tuition, regardless of their level of pre-college education. Others offered only classroom teaching, leaving students without any interaction with patients prior to graduation. Many new doctors were ill-prepared to care for the sick and had to learn by experience. Such schools were lucrative financial enterprises, and they turned out more doctors than the population required, creating competition between physicians for patients. Other schools required more stringent entry criteria, limited their enrollment in order to match the numbers of graduates to the needs of the community, collaborated with local hospitals to create a hands-on teaching environment, and coupled scientific research with the medical school curriculum. Johns Hopkins was the first American medical school to impose a four-year curriculum, in 1893. The university also required students to have completed four years of college before starting medical school. Many medical schools followed suit, but others did not, so by the early 1900s a wide variety of schools and standards existed.

In 1906, the American Medical Association (AMA) commissioned a study of medical schools in the United States. Its conclusion was that "too many poorly trained doctors were being turned out by substandard medical schools."[1] These included schools of osteopathy, chiropractic, and homeopathy. Subsequently, the Carnegie Foundation sent an educator, Abraham Flexner, and a representative of the AMA to inspect all 131 medical schools in the United States and Canada. Flexner and his colleagues gave an exhaustive account of each school, reporting on the entrance requirements, number of students in attendance, number of teaching staff and their qualifications, resources available for maintenance, the state of the laboratory facilities, and whether there were clinical facilities (meaning whether students had access to a clinic or hospital where they could be involved in patient care).[2]

---

1. John Abramson, MD, *Overdosed America: The Broken Promise of American Medicine* (New York: Harper Collins, 2004), 196.

2. Abraham Flexner, *Medical Education in the United States and Canada: A Report to the Carnegie Foundation for the Advancement of Teaching* (New York: Carnegie Foundation, 1910), http://archive.carnegiefoundation.org/pdfs/elibrary/Carnegie_Flexner_Report.pdf.

When the Flexner report was released in 1910, it recommended that all but thirty-one of the 131 schools be closed because of "an enormous over-production of uneducated and ill trained medical practitioners" and "an absolute disregard of the public welfare."[3] This "reconstruction" of the medical education system, as Flexner called it, aimed to improve the quality of medical schools and graduating physicians while creating a sustainable doctor-to-patient ratio that would meet the needs of the public.

Even though approximately one-half of the schools survived, the number of graduating students was cut by half. Some say this was the primary intent of the AMA, resulting in less competition for its members from other sorts of physicians. An in-depth examination of this era can be found in Paul Starr's book *The Social Transformation of American Medicine* (Basic Books, 1982). He notes that this shift encouraged the predominance of the physician-scientist, and the previously practical emphasis in American medicine was cast aside.

After the Flexner report was released, the vast majority of the funding given for university-based medical research came from the Carnegie and Rockefeller Foundations. This further encouraged an inclination toward scientific research, and that research became a key factor in the standing of the schools. As Dr. Abramson points out in *Overdosed America*, it also "set the stage for what evolved into the growing synergy between universities, the pharmaceutical and other medical industries."[4]

Not all medical doctors received the Flexner report enthusiastically. Even though Flexner did champion clinical hands-on training, some felt the emphasis on science predominated, leaving little room for the art of medicine. Sir William Osler had been the first professor of medicine at Johns Hopkins and, at the time of the release of the Flexner report, was a professor of medicine at Oxford, in England. He had a huge influence on medical education. Like Flexner, Dr. Osler felt it was important for

---

3. Ibid, x.

4. John Abramson, MD, *Overdosed America: The Broken Promise of American Medicine* (New York: Harper Collins, 2004), 197.

medical students to learn at the bedside. So, early in their academic training, his students were interviewing and examining hospitalized patients. Even such distinguished clinicians as Sir William Osler had serious concerns over the report and its interpretation, which seemed to favor science over humanism in medicine. Abraham Flexner himself felt that the strict scientific inclination of medical education suppressed the resourcefulness and humanity of the students.[5]

Over the past one hundred years, the format for American medical education has continued in the same vein. Before being admitted to medical school, one must complete a four-year college degree. Medical school is still a four-year curriculum, followed by a combination of internship and residency that can last anywhere from three to five years depending on the specialty. It is during internship and residency that young doctors essentially apprentice in their chosen field of medicine. Following residency, a great many doctors go on to do a fellowship and become subspecialists. For example, after completing a residency in internal medicine, one could go on to do a fellowship to become a cardiologist or intensive care specialist or dermatologist or endocrinologist. A gynecologist could do a fellowship in gynecologic oncology (gynecologic cancers), maternal-fetal medicine (high-risk pregnancy), or reproductive endocrinology. Someone who finishes a residency in family medicine can go on to do extra training in emergency medicine, obstetrics, or gerontology. There seems to be no end to the amount of training one could do.

Throughout these dozen or more years, students of medicine at every stage find themselves within a strictly hierarchical system. More senior and, therefore, more experienced doctors supervise the junior, less experienced ones. The hours of work have become slightly less grueling than they were even twenty years ago, when being on call day after day

---

5. Ibid.; Edmund D. Pelligrino, MD, "The Reconciliation between Technology and Humanism: A Flexnerian Task 75 Years Later," in *Flexner: 75 Years Later: A Current Commentary on Medical Education*, ed. Charles Vevier (Lanham, MD: University Press of America, 1987), 77.

was common. Now, in most states, interns may not work more than fourteen hours in a day. Still, fatigue and sleep deprivation are the norm. Over the years, novice physicians emerge at the other end of their training with an appreciation of the complexity of human beings and the skills with which to treat them. (For a superb account of this process, we highly recommend the book *Complications: A Surgeon's Notes on an Imperfect Science*, by Dr. Atul Gawande, Henry Holt, 2002.)

For the most part, the basis of these skills and experience has been derived from the Western biomedical model. This is the idea that the underlying cause of a disease can be found at the most minute level of function, which could be at the cellular level or even lower, such as the genetic or molecular level. It is remarkable to think that the failure of a few molecules to link in a normal way can cause a devastating disease. Unfortunately, this can be true of many illnesses, because molecular dysfunction can lead to abnormalities at increasingly higher levels of physiologic activities. Following the biomedical model, one would then try to devise high-tech treatments to correct the underlying problem at the cellular, genetic, or molecular level.

The problem with this model is that it focuses on the minute mechanism but overlooks the possibility of interplay between many factors that can contribute to a disease. These factors can be specific to an individual, like genetics, family environment, and personal life experiences, or they can affect the community at large, like environmental pollution, food additives, and poor access to markets with fresh produce or green spaces in which to exercise.

The dynamics of the origin of disease are highly complex, especially with respect to the chronic diseases of Western societies. In fact, even though the biomedical model claims to have found the root cause of an illness, many examples show that correcting what is thought to be the root cause with medication is not as effective as lifestyle changes. For example, elevated cholesterol (specifically, low-density lipoproteins, also known as LDL) is thought to cause cardiovascular disease by clogging arteries and leading to heart attacks. The "cure" in this instance is thought to be the use of statin medications that lower LDL and total cholesterol. However, several studies have shown that interventions such as exercise, dietary changes, and smoking-cessation counseling result in fewer deaths from coronary artery disease than do statin medications. The Lyon Diet Heart Study was one of the first studies of the anti-inflammatory Mediterranean diet. It showed that adherence to this diet decreased the risk of death even when cholesterol and LDL levels remained unchanged.[6]

This demonstrates that the biomedical model may not be the best way to institute effective medical care. Perhaps it is in everyone's best interest that doctors take a wider view of health and illness. Yes, it may be true that biochemical changes may increase the risk of certain diseases. For example, it is now scientifically proven that the chemicals released while the body is under stress lead to chronic inflammation and a higher risk of many conditions such as heart disease and cancer. But the more important question is, why doesn't everyone exposed to such stresses develop these diseases? Some people live under enormous physical and emotional strain, yet they do not succumb to these illnesses. What is it about the way they handle stress, the way their body heals, and their daily routines that sets them apart from their less fortunate neighbors?

These are not questions that Western physicians are trained to ask or investigate beyond mere lip service. But we feel that the biomedical model does not apply uniformly and exclusively to patient care. Sir William Osler is often quoted in this regard, saying, "It is much more important to know what sort of a patient has a disease than what sort of a disease a patient has."

Happily, starting at the end of the twentieth century, there has been a shift in the teachings of Western medicine. Increasingly, students of

---

6. John Abramson, MD, *Overdosed America: The Broken Promise of American Medicine* (New York: Harper Collins, 2004), 201; M. de Lorgeril, P. Salen, J. L. Martin, I. Monjaud, J. Delaye, and N. Mamelle, "Mediterranean Diet, Traditional Risk Factors, and the Rate of Cardiovascular Complications after Myocardial Infarction: Final Report of the Lyon Diet Heart Study," *Circulation* 99 (6): 779–785.

Western biomedicine are being trained to consider all aspects of individuals and their illnesses, such that the field of "biopsychosocial" medicine has evolved. Biopsychosocial medicine evaluates not just the biological cause of a disease but also the psychological, emotional, spiritual, and socioeconomic factors involved. All these added factors can both affect and be affected by the disease process. This biopsychosocial focus keeps the medical process patient-centered, rather than disease-centered.

Additionally, medical students are being exposed to complementary and alternative therapies and are instructed on ways to incorporate these therapies into a patient's plan of care. In fact, a number of North America's most prestigious medical schools now have departments of integrative medicine, which incorporate biomedicine with other modalities such as Eastern medicine, homeopathy, naturopathy, Western herbology, bodywork, mind-body medicine, and energetic therapies. Increasingly, Western physicians are open to learning about and utilizing these complementary techniques in order to improve the lives of their patients.

The History and Philosophy of Eastern Medicine

Before discussing the chronology of Eastern medicine, an understanding of its philosophy is extremely important. The principles of Eastern medicine hinge on the concept that man is inseparable from the universe. This notion comes from the observations and practices of Daoism. Having at least a minimal understanding of Daoism is essential for appreciating the theories of Eastern medicine.

Daoism is a philosophical system that was reportedly founded by Laozi (b. 604 BCE). While Laozi formulated the tenets of Daoism, it was his students and followers who wrote the majority of the formal texts that are the foundation of this philosophy. Prior to the advent of Daoism in China, as in every primitive civilization, the ancients observed the changes that took place over time in the world around them. They noted the cycles of the moon, planets, and stars. These celestial patterns were correlated to weather changes, growing seasons, and animal migrations.

Daoism grew out of this naturalist school of thought as it attempted to understand man's place in the order of the universe. This law of nature is called "the Dao" or "the Path." The Dao represents the basic principles from which all phenomena follow, including all aspects of human behavior.

In addition to the ideas of the Dao and the phases in the physical world that change over time, Daoist thinkers helped formalize the concept of the unity of opposites within nature. This is the basis of yin-yang theory, for which Eastern medicine is known. By starting with the concept of opposition to describe the relationship between two entities, Daoists formulated a dynamic view of the world that could be used to explain universal processes. A classic example of this mode of thought is the observation that there is always a sunny side and a shady side to a hill: one can say this side of the hill is sunny only by comparing it to the shady side. Labels are given to each item, described as either yin or yang, depending on its degree of substantiality. If something is more substantial in nature, it is yin. If it is more ethereal, it is yang. But these definitions have meaning only when compared one to the other. Any of the pairs that embody yin and yang cannot be separated and are not absolute.

The yin-yang experience is a fundamental factor in the development of the Daoist metaphysic. Far from designating yang as "something" and yin as "nothing," Daoism recognizes that both are active and that one creates the other.[7]

> Clay is molded into vessels,
> And because of the space where nothing exists we are able to
>   use them as vessels.
> Doors and windows are cut out in the walls of a house
> And because they are empty space, we are able to use them.
>   —Laozi (attributed)
>   from the *Dao De Ching*
>   (*The Classic of Dao and Virtue*)

---

7. Michael M. Zanoni, PhD, conversation with author (CK), April 10, 2011.

From this thought arises the realization that the part and whole must exist simultaneously. The infinite exists at every singular point in space, and eternity is found in every individual moment. The Daoist consideration of the infinite and the yin-yang experience infuses itself into the practice of Eastern medicine by virtue of the fact that dysfunction within the patient, known as the pattern of disharmony, cannot be viewed separately from the patient. The part and whole exist together and define each other.

In addition to the concepts of Dao and yin-yang, the recognition of the phases of the universe developed into the theory known as Wu Xing, or Five Phases. These phases or elements are known as water, wood, fire, earth, and metal.

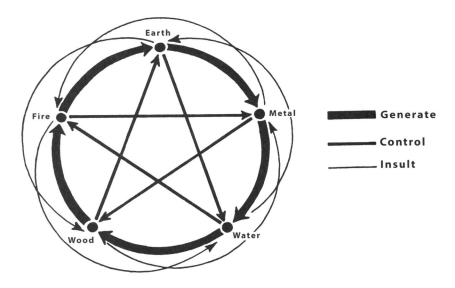

This doctrine of "systematic correspondences" was used to understand and interrelate naturally occurring phenomena and apply this understanding to medicine, as well as other disciplines, including astrology, social politics, and natural sciences.[8] Using this paradigm, Daoist

---

8. Joseph Helms, MD, *Acupuncture Energetics: A Clinical Approach for Physicians* (Berkeley, CA: Medical Acupuncture Publishers, 1995), 17.

physicians looked at the human body as a microcosm of the universe and sought to use the natural laws of the universe to maintain a harmonious balance. They acknowledged that this balance must occur internally and also with the patient's external environment. Following the principles of Daoism, which emphasize moderation and equilibrium, the patient would be cautioned to follow the middle path in all aspects of life: to rest but also exercise, to work but have time for leisure, to eat a variety of healthy foods but neither too much nor too little. By achieving this equilibrium, the movement of the intelligent vital force within the body (called qi) would be smooth. This free movement of qi would maintain optimal health.

In 1973, in the Chinese province of Hunan, a famous archeological dig discovered silk scrolls that discussed subjects as diverse as astrology, art, military strategy, philosophy, and medicine. There were even two copies of Laozi's *Dao De Ching*. These scrolls were found in the Mawangdui tombs (King Ma's Mound). Scientific methods were used to date the scrolls from approximately 200 BCE, and the tomb itself had been sealed in 168 BCE. The medical texts from these scrolls cover physiology, illness, surgery, herbal treatments, and what has been translated as macrobiotic hygiene. Macrobiotic hygiene involves not only the body but also the spirit. This section discusses longevity, sexuality, and diet. Breathing and physical exercises are recommended to treat illness and cultivate health. There are also writings on magic and incantations.[9]

Illness is described in the Mawangdui medical manuscripts as the result of a disturbance in the movement of qi within the eleven vessels of the body. These vessels that contain qi are different than the arteries and veins that contain blood. The treatment that was advocated at the time involved cauterization of the qi vessels. There is no mention of using acupuncture needles to correct the flow of qi. Instead, the medical practitioners who wrote these manuscripts advocated the use of food,

---

9. Donald J. Harper, *Early Chinese Medical Literature: The Mawangdui Medical Manuscripts* (London: Routledge, Taylor, and Francis, 1998), 6.

herbs, breath control, and exercise to improve the flow of qi and achieve a long and vibrant life.

This approach to good health was formalized in the classic medical text of the Han dynasty (206 BCE–220 CE), the *Huang Di Nei Jing* (*The Yellow Emperor's Classic of Internal Medicine*). It is thought that this text is a compilation of medical writings from practitioners of earlier centuries. It takes the form of a discussion between the Yellow Emperor (Huang Di) and his minister and is significant in that it was the first known text to move away from shamanism and supernatural causes of disease. Like the Mawangdui medical manuscripts, the *Huang Di Nei Jing* discussed the prevention and treatment of illness through diet, exercise, and herbs. Acupuncture theory is well described in the second volume of this text. The principles of energy flow within the body (qi), yin-yang theory, and diagnostic techniques are also discussed.

Around the first century BCE, the art of acupuncture using metal needles was formalized. Some researchers of Chinese medical history state that acupuncture arose from the practice of using sharpened stones and bones to lance infected skin, allowing the body to heal. However, scholars such as Paul Unschuld and Donald Harper state that the vessel theory and treatment paradigm delineated in the Mawangdui medical manuscripts was the necessary precursor to acupuncture theory, as described in the *Huang Di Nei Jing*.[10]

Through trial and error, the Chinese determined that placing acupuncture needles at specific sites would give consistent and reproducible results. By the time the *Huang Di Nei Jing* was written, the intricate system of acupuncture points and qi flow within acupuncture channels was well established. Twelve paired principal channels, or vessels, were described, meaning that the channels were duplicated on each side of the body in a mirror image. These paired channels are named for organs of the body. The channels are kidney, heart, small intestine,

10. Ibid., 5.

The Body Channels

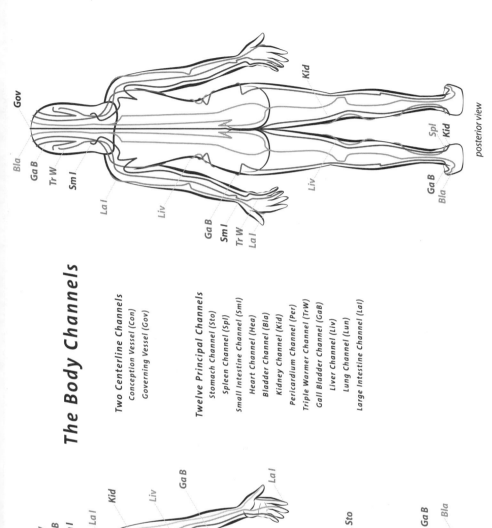

Two Centerline Channels
Conception Vessel (Con)
Governing Vessel (Gov)

Twelve Principal Channels
Stomach Channel (Sto)
Spleen Channel (Spl)
Small Intestine Channel (SmI)
Heart Channel (Hea)
Bladder Channel (Bla)
Kidney Channel (Kid)
Pericardium Channel (Per)
Triple Warmer Channel (TrW)
Gall Bladder Channel (GaB)
Liver Channel (Liv)
Lung Channel (Lun)
Large Intestine Channel (LaI)

anterior view

posterior view

Illustration courtesy of Shutterstock

urinary bladder, spleen, lung, large intestine, stomach, liver, *san jiao*,[11] pericardium,[12] and gallbladder.

While the channels can directly influence the named organ, they also affect other areas and physiological processes. Additionally, eight "extraordinary" channels were noted. These special channels run in various directions, over and through the body, connecting the principal channels and acting as reservoirs of qi. Acupuncture theory is discussed in more detail later in this chapter.

As in all ancient civilizations, the Chinese used indigenous plants, minerals, and animals as medicine. Chinese herbology predates acupuncture, probably by thousands of years, but until the development of written language, the use of these medicinals was not documented. Several very famous texts categorize Chinese herbs and explain their function. *Shen Nong Ben Cao Jing* (*The Divine Farmer's Materia Medica*) was written in the early Tang dynasty (452–536 CE), but it is actually a compilation of much earlier writings. The book discusses the attributes of 365 herbs, the majority of which are still used today.

Dr. Zhang Zhong Jin (150–219 CE) was renowned for his text, the *Shang Han Lun* (*Treatise on Cold Damage*). This is the oldest formulary to group patient symptoms into clinically useful categories. Zhang Zhong Jin was also the first to link diagnoses derived through the principles of yin-yang theory and the Wu Xing (Five Phases) with standardized herbal treatments.

One of the most celebrated physicians in the history of Chinese medicine was Dr. Li Shi Zhen. He lived during the Ming dynasty and in 1578 wrote his masterpiece, the *Ben Cao Gang Mu* (*Compendium of Materia Medica*). Li Shi Zhen traveled across China in search of medicinal herbs. After twenty-seven years of diligent work, the *Ben Cao Gang Mu* was completed. It documents 1,892 distinct herbs and over eleven thousand formulas. This comprehensive text remained the official materia medica for China for the next four hundred years.

---

11. Also known as Triple Heater or Triple Burner.
12. Also known as Master of the Heart.

Two other noteworthy Chinese doctors are Hua Tuo (145–203 CE) and Sun Si-Miao (581–683 CE). Hua Tuo was well known, especially for his surgical skills and the development of a particular type of exercise that he called Five Animal Play (Wu Qin Xi). Sun Si-Miao stood out not only for talent as a healer, but also for his humanity. Although the emperors of the Tang dynasty wanted Sun Si-Miao as the palace physician, he declined and worked for all people. In his writings, he instructed doctors to be of good moral character and to treat all patients equally regardless of their class or wealth.

Around the time of Sun Si-Miao, during the fifth and sixth centuries, Eastern medicine spread from China to Japan, Korea, and Vietnam. Through trade via the Silk Road, knowledge of this system of medicine eventually arrived in the Middle East and Europe, with little more than passing interest outside of Asia until much later. As European colonization of East Asia increased, more Western physicians became curious about these techniques. France had colonized Vietnam, and so French physicians who traveled there were exposed to the successes of acupuncture and herbal formulas. From the eighteenth century onward, the French were at the forefront of Western investigations of Eastern medicine. Later in this chapter, we discuss the science of acupuncture in greater detail.

Eastern Medicine in America

An increasing percentage of the general population has benefited from Eastern medicine over the past half century, but very few were able to take advantage of this powerful medical system prior to the 1970s. Until then, acupuncture was illegal in the United States. Even though it was utilized and well respected throughout Europe, Britain, Canada, Japan, and other Asian countries, both practitioners and patients who sought to use this medicine risked arrest in the United States. For this reason, there is very little documentation of the early history of Eastern medicine in America. There are, however, some accounts dating as far back as the nineteenth century.

In 1887, the Chinese immigrants Ing Hay and Lung On arrived in Oregon to work as miners. Because foreign workers had little access to doctors, Hay and On soon started to treat their fellow countrymen using their knowledge of Chinese medicine. After word spread of the excellent remedies that Hay and On provided, the townsfolk also sought out their care.

During the next eighty years or so, Chinese medicine remained an underground endeavor. In every Chinatown throughout the United States, practitioners of acupuncture would secretly treat patients in back rooms and condemned buildings. One such patient was Barbara Bernie. Ms. Bernie was an American architecture and design consultant who sought to use Chinese medicine to alleviate her chronic fatigue syndrome. She ended up going to Canada for treatment, then subsequently studied traditional Chinese medicine with the famed Dr. John Worsley in the United Kingdom.

After completing her studies in 1971, Ms. Bernie returned to the United States and began to champion the cause of Chinese medicine. She invited Dr. Worsley to speak in America regarding the benefits of this healing system. In 1973, she met Dr. Miriam Lee, and together they worked to change the legal status of acupuncture in California.[13]

Dr. Lee was born in China and was a trained midwife and acupuncturist. When she came to America in 1966, she could not practice her chosen profession, so she worked in a factory. Gradually, however, she saw the need within her community and started to practice acupuncture in secrecy. By 1972, the practice of acupuncture was permitted in California only under particular circumstances. The state of California allowed non-physician, unlicensed practitioners to practice acupuncture under the direct supervision of a licensed doctor, only if the procedure was performed in an approved medical school and only if the purpose of the treatment was for scientific research. Clearly, these

---

13. July 16, 2004, http://www.sfgate.com/news/article/BERNIE-Barbara-2741262.php.

restrictions were a long way from the autonomous practice that acupuncturists enjoyed in a large part of the rest of the world.

In 1974, Nevada and Oregon became the first states to legalize the practice of acupuncture, but it was still illegal in California, where Miriam Lee and Barbara Bernie were treating patients surreptitiously. In 1974, Dr. Lee was arrested for practicing medicine without a license. During her trial, hundreds of Dr. Lee's patients rallied to support her and crowded the courtroom to testify on her behalf.[14] After the trial, then governor Ronald Reagan designated acupuncture as an experimental procedure. In 1976, thanks to the persistent work of Miriam Lee, Barbara Bernie, and some state senators, a bill was passed that legalized acupuncture in California. Certificates to practice were then issued to qualified individuals. By 1979, California deleted the original requirements of the 1976 bill, which stipulated that a patient must be referred by a medical doctor, dentist, podiatrist, or chiropractor in order to receive acupuncture treatments.

Since 1974, the vast majority of states have legalized acupuncture, though some, like Alabama, only allow medical doctors, osteopaths, and chiropractors to practice this technique. Interestingly, Alabama and some other states may not require these health-care providers to have any formal training in acupuncture prior to treating patients with this modality. This, however, is not the case in most states (we discuss the training requirements for Western medical personnel to practice acupuncture below).

During the 1980s, various organizations were created to ensure national standards within the profession. These included the National Commission for the Certification of Acupuncturists, which set benchmarks for safe and competent practice. In later years, this became the National Certification Commission for Acupuncture and Oriental

---

14. Laurel Skurko Koa, "Legalizing Acupuncture in California," http://www.healthy.net/Health/Essay/Legalizing_Acupuncture_in_California/50/1 (accessed January 2, 2014).

Medicine (NCCAOM). By including Oriental medicine, criteria could also be set for other modalities within Eastern medicine, such as herbology and the style of bodywork known as *tui na*.

In 1988, the US Department of Education approved the Accreditation Commission for Acupuncture and Oriental Medicine (ACAOM). The ACAOM is the organization authorized to accredit master's level programs in acupuncture schools in the United States. In 1992, schools of Oriental medicine were subject to review by the ACAOM and, in 2011, the scope of the ACAOM was increased to include accreditation of postgraduate doctoral level programs in acupuncture and Oriental medicine.[15] Though a postgraduate doctoral degree is not currently required to practice acupuncture and Oriental medicine, more American schools are becoming accredited and offering advanced training to those who desire it.

Standards for both entry-level educational prerequisites and hours of training needed to graduate have increased over time. While rules vary from state to state, the most stringent criteria require a four-year baccalaureate degree prior to acceptance to a school of Oriental medicine. This is the same sort of prerequisite demanded for entry to a Western medical school. The master of science of Oriental medicine (MSOM) degree is a four-year endeavor, demanding as much as 3,300 hours of training. After obtaining an MSOM degree, a candidate may sit for the NCCAOM certification examinations. Having passed the exams, the candidate becomes a certified diplomate. These exams must be passed in order to apply for a license to practice acupuncture and Oriental medicine. After graduating from school, passing the boards, and being issued a license, the practitioner becomes a licensed acupuncturist (LAc). This is equivalent to the process a Western physician must undergo. Simply finishing medical school is insufficient to obtain a license to practice medicine. Every medical school graduate must pass the United States Medical Licensing Exam (USMLE), then qualify for a state medical license in order to be licensed to treat patients. A graduate

---

15. www.acaom.org.

of a school of acupuncture and Oriental medicine is subject to a similar rigorous standard.

Meanwhile, the value of acupuncture has not escaped the notice of Western-trained American physicians. One particular such physician is Dr. Joseph Helms. Dr. Helms is a graduate of Johns Hopkins University and the UCLA School of Medicine. Dr. Helms completed his acupuncture training in France and has been teaching acupuncture to physicians since 1977. He went on to offer the first course on medical acupuncture for physicians in the United States in 1980 and founded the American Academy of Medical Acupuncturists (AAMA). From 1982 to 2008, Dr. Helms and the instructors of the Helms Medical Institute (HMI) taught courses in medical acupuncture under the sponsorship of the continuing medical education departments of the UCLA and Stanford schools of medicine. In 2008, the Helms Medical Institute was accredited by the Accreditation Council for Continuing Medical Education as the sole sponsor of the HMI courses.[16] Since its inception, HMI and Dr. Helms have trained over six thousand physician acupuncturists. These graduates must pass an exam administered by the American Board of Medical Acupuncturists (ABMA) in order to become certified.

There are differences between a medical or physician acupuncturist and a licensed acupuncturist. A medical acupuncturist is a physician (either medical doctor or doctor of osteopathy) who has completed the minimum number of hours of acupuncture training required by their home state. This can vary widely by state, but usually between 220 and 300 hours of training are mandatory. The physician layers the study of acupuncture on top of an already extensive knowledge of Western medicine and clinical acumen; however, there may be little formal training in Chinese herbology.

In contrast, a licensed acupuncturist devotes approximately ten times that number of hours to training in both acupuncture and herbology, as well as *tui na* and other Chinese therapeutic modalities. Many hundreds of hours of Western biomedicine are included in the

---

16. Helms Medical Institute, http://www.hmieducation.com.

curriculum. This includes biology, chemistry, human anatomy, physiology, pathophysiology, and pharmacology. While a medical acupuncturist must be a doctor first, a licensed acupuncturist need not be. It is interesting to note that many medical acupuncturists seek out more training in Eastern medicine and enroll in master's-level programs in Oriental medicine, eventually becoming licensed acupuncturists.

The mark of an excellent practitioner, whether a medical or licensed acupuncturist, is the willingness to refine the art of Eastern medicine. This is done by attending specialized courses and lectures, engaging in private reading, and striving to perfect one's technique. As medical care in America becomes more integrated, a patient may encounter either type of acupuncturist in the clinic or hospital setting. In fact, many hospitals now have departments of acupuncture with both licensed and medical acupuncturists working side by side for the greater benefit of the patient.

The Science of Acupuncture: An East-West Fusion

From China to Europe to the rest of the world, interest in and use of Chinese medicine has grown during the past century, surging over the last fifty years. The concept of using plants as medicines was well established in Europe, as it was throughout the world, but it was the mystery of acupuncture that fascinated the French. This led to various scientific experiments that laid the foundation for modern acupuncture research.

During the mid-twentieth century, the French and the Chinese performed a number of experiments that began to explain how acupuncture works. There is no single, simple explanation for acupuncture's mechanism of action. Each scientist added new information, helping to fill in the pieces of the puzzle.

In the 1940s and 1950s, Niboyet designed a series of experiments that showed electrical resistance is lower at acupuncture points than elsewhere on the body. This means electricity will pass into the body more easily across the skin at an acupuncture point than across the skin at a non-acupuncture point. Niboyet also demonstrated that electricity flowed more easily along the same acupuncture channel than between channels that were not as strongly related to each other. These results were confirmed by other scientists in the 1960s and 1970s.[17]

The acupuncture channel itself has remained an elusive entity. Our understanding of acupuncture channels and how acupuncture works has changed over time. Acupuncture channels are intimately associated with the neural, immune, and endocrine systems of the body. For example, modern acupuncture researchers note the channels that run on the inner arms almost exactly follow the paths of the nerves. Though the ancient Chinese were aware of the existence of the structures we call nerves, they did not know their function. They could not have known that electrical signals travel along nerves, having no knowledge of electricity.

Understanding that the effect of acupuncture is mediated via electricity was the first step in uncovering its mechanism of action. Over the past half century, the unfolding of this knowledge began by seeking evidence that these channels do exist. They were thought to be different from the known vascular or neurological systems that have been defined by modern medicine. The first piece of indirect evidence of the existence of acupuncture channels is that many patients experience a feeling of heaviness, achiness, or warmth around the acupuncture needles during treatments. These sensations can radiate from the needles, either circumferentially or linearly. When moving linearly, this feeling of warmth or achiness travels up or down the area of the body being needled. Modern Chinese researchers define this phenomenon by the term "propagated sensation along channels."[18] They suggest that this sensation represents the movement of a corrective signal to an area determined by the acupuncture point that has been used. The target zone for the propagated sensation need not be a local area. An example of a

---

17. Joseph Helms, MD, *Acupuncture Energetics: A Clinical Approach for Physicians* (Berkeley, CA: Medical Acupuncture Publishers, 1995), 21.
18. Ibid., 22.

response in a distant organ is seen in the following study. Patients were needled at a point along the stomach channel while the activity of their stomachs was observed using radiographic imaging. Some patients reported feeling this propagated sensation reach their stomachs and others did not. In those patients who felt the sensation, the radiographic images demonstrated stronger but less frequent gastric muscle contractions than those who had no sensation at all.[19] We now know that the sensations elicited by acupuncture are caused by the activation of different types of nerve fibers.[20]

The speed of the propagated sensation has been noted to travel at one to ten centimeters per second. This velocity varies among subjects and with the intensity of the needling. This rate is much, much slower than the speed of nerve impulses, so it cannot be attributed simply to nerve conduction. The brain itself may also be involved in the perception of this sensation. Some studies have reported that amputees who are aware of phantom limbs are able to feel the propagated sensation within the absent limb when needled along a channel associated with the limb in question. This indicates that there must be some central nervous system involvement in the appreciation of this sensation.

The second piece of indirect evidence involves numerous experiments performed by the French researcher Mussat, demonstrating differences in propagation of electricity along acupuncture channels versus areas of the body not classically described as being on acupuncture channels. He consistently found that electrical resistance between two acupuncture points on the same channel was less than that found between two non-acupuncture points in the same vicinity. Through his other experiments, Mussat discovered that the electrical signal traveled through the body at a speed of approximately 1.7 centimeters per second and that electrical current passes through acupuncture channels in an organized fashion, through networks described by the ancient Chinese.

---

19. Ibid.

20. Michael Corradino, *Neuropuncture: A Clinical Handbook of Neuroscience Acupuncture*, 2nd ed. (London: Singing Dragon, 2013), 24.

Although the acupuncture channels cannot be physically identified either with the naked eye or under a microscope, acupuncture points have been examined extensively. Researchers Bossy, Senelar, and Auziech separately studied the composition of acupuncture points. They biopsied acupuncture points from both animals and humans, examined them microscopically, and made a number of discoveries.[21]

Bossy noted that acupuncture points measure from one to five square millimeters in size, and the majority of the points are located between muscles. Senelar described the microscopic appearance of biopsied acupuncture points as having a particular configuration. The individual parts of the point were not unusual; he saw blood vessels, nerves, lymphatics, and fibrous tissue connecting the layers of the skin. What was different was the way these components were arranged within the area of the acupuncture point. The fibrous connective tissue was looser than that of the surrounding skin. This accounts for the palpable sponginess of many acupuncture points. It also makes the point a better electrical conductor. The acupuncture point was aligned in a vertical fashion, as though creating a conduit from the surface of the skin to deeper tissues. Within the loose connective tissue was a lymphatic core, partnered with an arteriole and vein, all of which traveled vertically up toward the skin.

Auziech found that the skin actually thins out over the acupuncture point, and Senelar stated that 80 percent of acupuncture points have the configuration as described above.[22] Electron microscopy has demonstrated a large concentration of tiny blood vessels and nerve endings within the column.

When an acupuncture point is needled, a lot happens on the cellular level. There seems to be another mechanism at play, aside from direct activation of the nervous system. When the needle is inserted, it is manipulated to create sensation. This manipulation causes a mechanical

---

21. Joseph Helms, MD, *Acupuncture Energetics: A Clinical Approach for Physicians* (Berkeley, CA: Medical Acupuncture Publishers, 1995), 26.
22. Ibid., 27.

change in the tissue. Researchers have demonstrated, using magnetic resonance imaging and ultrasound elastography, that a slow-moving wave is generated through the tissue that has been needled. There is also a shift in calcium ions that creates a biochemical signal that appears to be separate from the electrical signal of the nerve fibers.[23]

Western science has added a great deal of supporting evidence for the existence of a communication network from acupuncture points to the rest of the body by documenting the effects of acupuncture on blood chemistry, body temperature, and hormone levels.

With respect to blood chemistry, acupuncture has been shown to modify levels of glucose, cortisol, triglycerides, and cholesterol. In the case of glucose, Omura demonstrated that blood glucose increased following acupuncture when the patients' pretreatment level was normal or low; however, when the pretreatment level was high, acupuncture caused glucose levels to decrease to normal values.[24] Although the mechanism of action is not well understood, acupuncture seems to assist the body in achieving balance. In medicine, this equilibrium is called homeostasis.

Acupuncture has also been shown to cause an increase in the body's surface temperature. This is caused by the dilation of vessels, resulting in increased blood flow. The increase has been documented at a rate three times higher than pretreatment flow. Not only does the surface temperature of the needled skin increase locally, but it also increases at the same area on the other side of the body.[25] Increased blood flow improves oxygenation within the tissue and may speed healing.

A great deal of research has been performed regarding acupuncture's effect on hormone and neurotransmitter levels, particularly with respect to pain relief. Some of these neurotransmitters include serotonin,

---

23. Edward S. Yang et al., "Ancient Chinese Medicine and Mechanistic Evidence of Acupuncture Physiology," *European Journal of Physiology* 462 (2011): 645–653, doi:10.1007/s00424-011-1017-3.

24. Joseph Helms, MD, *Acupuncture Energetics: A Clinical Approach for Physicians* (Berkeley, CA: Medical Acupuncture Publishers, 1995), 41.

25. Ibid., 40.

norepinephrine, substance P, GABA (gamma-aminobutyric acid), and dopamine. All of these compounds work together to diminish the brain's perception of pain.

Another way in which pain is decreased is through the release of cortisol, which has an anti-inflammatory action. The release of cortisol is controlled by levels of adrenocorticotrophic hormone (ACTH), and acupuncture has been shown to increase the discharge of this substance.

Also, acupuncture modulates the body's internal production of opioids, leading to pain relief through a different pathway. Opioids are narcotic-like compounds; those produced in the body are called endorphins, which attach to receptors located on cell membranes, resulting in decreased pain. Endorphins comprise several different types, and each acts at a different site within the brain and spinal cord to relieve pain. Interestingly, it appears that certain endorphins (beta-endorphin and met-enkephalin) also interact with the immune system. A surge in the levels of these endorphins can lead to increased activity of natural killer cells, a type of white blood cell that defends the body from foreign microbes and cancerous mutations.[26]

For all the various effects that acupuncture produces, the specific mechanism of action has not yet been completely discovered. As we have seen, electricity is a principal mediator of information that is passed along through the body, creating numerous physiologic changes.

Several theories exist regarding the ways in which these processes are regulated. Most of them concentrate on the effects produced by the passage of electrical current through the body. There is no doubt that the human body utilizes electricity in its everyday functioning. Western medicine has used this information to create many diagnostic tests and therapies.

In the heart, the interpretation of the electrical signals seen on an electrocardiogram (EKG) allows a physician to diagnose a heart attack or cardiac rhythm disturbance. If a patient's heart suddenly stops beating,

---

26. Ibid., 41.

electricity is applied to the person's chest via a device called a defibrillator in an effort to "kick-start" cardiac activity. Smaller amounts of electricity are also used to change irregular rhythms to regular ones.

The electrical signals from the brain can be studied to help diagnose epilepsy or sleep disturbances. We can assess the health of these systems by recording the speed of electrical impulses through the nerves and muscles.

Even skin healing, which we tend to take for granted, requires electricity to activate the restorative process. Electrically, the skin can be described as a battery, with the negative charge inside each cell and the positive charge on the exterior surface. When the skin is breached, either by trauma or by inserting an acupuncture needle, the "battery" is short-circuited, and now the charge on the skin surface is negative. This negative charge seems to be an initiating factor in healing and activates the body's system of repair. It has been shown that this negative charge, described by Dr. Robert Becker as a "current of injury," can last several days following an acupuncture treatment.[27]

Dr. Becker, an American orthopedic surgeon, performed a fascinating series of experiments involving electrical current and limb regeneration in salamanders and frogs. Even though salamanders and frogs are closely related, salamanders can spontaneously regrow lost limbs, but frogs cannot. Through his research, Dr. Becker discovered that the tissue over the salamanders' limb stumps display a relatively negative charge compared with other points on the animal. The frogs did not exhibit this negative charge. When he applied the appropriate electrical current and created a negative charge over the area of the frogs' missing limbs, the frogs' limbs regenerated just like the salamanders' did.[28] Dr. Becker's work has led to the creation of electrical devices that accelerate bone healing. These devices are used in cases in which broken bones are not healing well. In the past, it was sometimes necessary to

---

27. Ibid., 67.

28. Richard Gerber, *Vibrational Medicine: The #1 Handbook of Subtle-Energy Therapies*, 3rd ed. (Rochester, VT: Bear and Company, 2001), 91.

amputate limbs that would not heal. By using electricity to enhance bone healing, Dr. Becker's discovery has decreased the need for amputation in such circumstances.

As well as the electrical component of the energy within the human body, there is also a magnetic constituent. Without this, magnetic resonance imaging (MRI) would not be possible. Studies called functional MRIs are used to observe the electromagnetic changes within different areas of the brain in response to acupuncture needling.

Other devices have been developed that can measure electromagnetic fields that come from diverse parts of the body. Such devices have demonstrated that electromagnetic fields exist around acupuncture points and that the intensity of these fields changes following acupuncture treatment.[29] Some researchers suggest that acupuncture points act as amplifiers by increasing the signal that moves along the channel.

Identifying the exact tissues through which these electromagnetic signals pass is a subject of ongoing study. Evidence suggests a variety of mechanisms through which bioelectrical information is transmitted. These mechanisms include the following:

- Electron-rich fluid that naturally bathes the tissues of the body organized into tiny pockets now recognized as the interstium, a newly defined organ[30]
- Perineural cells (cells that are adjacent to nerves)
- Proteins such as hormones and neurotransmitters that regulate communication between cells
- The fascia, a fibrous tissue that surrounds and connects every component of the body, from nerves, arteries, and veins to each muscle and organ

29. Joseph Helms, MD, *Acupuncture Energetics: A Clinical Approach for Physicians*, 1st ed. (Berkeley, CA: Medical Acupuncture Publishers, 1995), 62.

30. Petros C. Benias et al., "Structure and Distribution of an Unrecognized Interstitium in Human Tissues," *Scientific Reports*, Volume 8, Article number: 4947(2018) doi:10.1038/s41598-018-23062-6.

In his exceptional book *The Spark in the Machine,* Dr. Daniel Keown explains the role that fascia plays in the body, including its electrical properties. Fascia is composed of collagen. Collagen is a protein that accounts for 30 percent of the proteins in our body. Proteins are made of amino acids. In collagen fibers, these amino acids are arranged into three threads that twist around each other like three-stranded rope, lending incredible tensile strength to the tissues in which it is found. These include bones, ligaments, tendons, cartilage, arteries, and connective tissue. Just like it sounds, connective tissue connects and surrounds all our organs and muscles. Collagen even creates the lattice of the interstitium and interacts directly with the fluid inside these bundles, potentially allowing communication between body systems.[31]

Dr. Keown explains that, because of its molecular structure, collagen can act like a crystal and generate small currents of piezoelectricity when it undergoes mechanical stress. If a substance is piezoelectric, it will generate a change in electrical charge when it is compressed then returns to its original shape. We take advantage of piezoelectricity when we use pilot lights on a gas grill to create a spark, igniting the flame. Collagen is also a semiconductor. This means that collagen can conduct electricity, but not as well as metals such as copper. It can also act as an insulator, but not as well as glass. So, with every movement you make, your tendons, muscles, and bones undergo mechanical strain, and the collagen generates an electrical current. Collagen is an integral part of the fascia that connects the top of your head to the tip of your toes. Dr. Keown describes this as "an interconnected, living electrical web."[32]

When an acupuncture needle is inserted into the body, it makes contact with this "living electrical web." The acupuncturist will usually manipulate the needle until both the patient and the practitioner are aware of a certain sensation. The patient may feel an ache or a slight electrical zing at the insertion site, and this feeling may propagate along the

---

31. Ibid.

32. Daniel Keown, *The Spark in the Machine: How the Science of Acupuncture Explains the Mysteries of Western Medicine* (London: Singing Dragon, 2014), 21.

body part that is needled. The acupuncturist can feel this through the needle. This sensation is called "de qi," or "the arrival of the qi." Even if the needle is inserted into an area that is not classified as an acupuncture point or is not along the channel, this sensation may be felt. This is because the fascia wraps the whole body, not only along acupuncture channels. Just as the blood flows through large vessels and tiny capillaries, so too does piezoelectricity traverse the whole body.

Knowing about the "body electric," researchers have tried to explain the location of acupuncture channels and points, forming hypotheses regarding the way in which bioelectromagnetic information travels through the body. Zhang and Popp theorize that electromagnetic energy travels in waves. These waves bounce off the physical structures in the body such as bones, nerves, and skin, creating interference patterns, similar to the way waves of water reflect off the sides of a pool. As they change direction, the waves combine with others, creating higher waves, or canceling each other out. Zhang and Popp suggest that acupuncture points and channels occur at areas where bioelectromagnetic waves have combined to form new waves of higher amplitudes, and that acupuncture needles can be used to change the body's electromagnetic field.

There may not be one single path through which acupuncture needles influence the state of the body. The human body is a complex system, and it seems likely that the ways in which acupuncture affects it are manifold. Further research will shed light on this intriguing phenomenon. Even though the mechanism of action is not fully understood, we can still benefit from the positive physiologic changes that acupuncture produces.

Now that we have discussed the history and philosophy of Eastern and Western medicine, in the next chapter we focus on how each discipline understands the underlying mechanism of disease and how our modern lifestyle influences our health.

CHAPTER 2

Qi, the Dao, and Cell Biology

B OTH WESTERN AND EASTERN medical traditions base their definition of health on the correct functioning of bodily systems. In the Western paradigm, this is considered optimal cellular metabolism. In the Eastern model, this is considered the smooth flow of qi. Which concept is correct? They both are.

Ancient practitioners of both healing arts recognized that the strength and abundance of a person's vital force, or qi, was predictive of their state of health and longevity. It was also noted that within families, vitality or frailty could be passed from generation to generation. In Eastern medicine, the qi you receive from your parents is called "pre-heaven qi." In Western medicine, this would be considered your genetic constitution.

Either way you look at it, these are the cards you are dealt. But, it is the decisions you make during the game that influence the outcome. These decisions include what you eat, the quality of air you breathe, whether you exercise, how long you sleep, how you manage your stress, how you view your place within your family and society, and many other factors. The combination of all these elements dictates the quality of the physical, emotional, and spiritual resources that sustain you. This is "post-heaven qi," from an Eastern perspective, and much of it is within your control. This holds true from a Western point of view too. You received a particular set of chromosomes from your parents. Maybe some of them predispose you toward developing heart disease, diabetes, or cancer, but these conditions are not a certainty. How you choose to live your life actually alters gene expression and the lifespan of cells in your body.

How does this work? Most cells in your body have a nucleus, the control center of the cell. Within the nucleus are your chromosomes, which are composed of genes. Your genes are like a blueprint. From conception and throughout your life, your genes are copied to create new cells. The genes you carry determine your potential: for example, how tall you might be or how fast your metabolism is or whether you are more likely to develop a certain type of cancer. Many factors affect the expression of your genes, such as what you eat; your level of physical activity; your work hours; the psychological stress you experience; and whether you smoke, drink alcohol, or are exposed to environmental pollutants.[1]

Even the act of copying can affect your genes. Every time a cell divides and has to make a copy of the genes within the nucleus, a bit of the genetic material at the ends of the chromosomes is lost. Over time, if enough genetic material is lost, the cell cannot function properly and dies. Genetic material is made up of DNA (deoxyribonucleic acid). The DNA is composed of pairs of nucleotides. The order in which these nucleotides are put together determines whether the sequence contains information that can regulate growth, metabolism, and reproduction through the creation of proteins. This type of DNA is called "coding" DNA. However, the majority of DNA does not code in this fashion but, rather, acts like punctuation in a sentence. A comma or a period does not have meaning in and of itself, but the placement of a punctuation mark creates coherence within a sentence. The DNA patterns that serve this function are called noncoding sequences.

One such noncoding DNA sequence, called the telomere, is found at the ends of each chromosome. The telomeres protect the coding

---

1. Jorge Alejandro Alegria-Torres, Andrea Baccarelli, and Valentina Bollati, "Epigenetics and Lifestyle," *Epigenomics* 3 (3): 267–277, doi:10.2217/epi.11.22.

DNA from damage during cell replication. Telomeres and their associated enzyme, telomerase, were discovered in the 1980s by Drs. Elizabeth Blackburn, Carol Greider, and Jack Szostak, who share a Nobel Prize for their groundbreaking work. Dr. Blackburn likens the telomere to the plastic bits on the ends of your shoelaces that prevent the shoelace from fraying. During each chromosome replication, the telomere shortens and then is rebuilt by telomerase. This is how telomeres protect the essential information within your cells, and it seems that the longer your telomeres, the greater the buffer you have against cell death.

Subsequent research indicates that telomere length, both normal and abnormal, can be inherited. Short telomeres may increase a person's risk of chronic illness. Some studies also show that telomere length may be positively influenced by decreasing physical and psychological stress through exercise, adequate sleep, improved nutrition, mindfulness, meditation, and qigong.[2] Telomere length in organ donors and recipients has even been used as a marker to estimate the risk of acute organ rejection or failure.[3]

Just as vibrant pre-heaven and post-heaven qi can often predict good health, telomere length can be used as a marker of well-being. One might say that telomeres and telomerase are one possible scientific explanation of the concept of pre-heaven and post-heaven qi. One day, science may completely explain all the phenomena that ancient practitioners described through careful observation.

But before you start an internet search for a supplement that will increase your telomerase levels, a word of warning from Dr. Blackburn: cancer cells have the ability to turn on telomerase, maintain long telo-

2. Elizabeth Blackburn, PhD, and Elissa Epel, PhD, *The Telomere Effect: A Revolutionary Approach to Living Younger, Healthier, Longer* (New York: Grand Central Publishing, 2017).

3. Karolina Kloda, Leszek Domanski, and Artur Mierzecki, "Telomere Length Assessment for Prediction of Organ Transplantation Outcome: Future or Failure: A Review of the Literature," *Medical Science Monitor* 23 (2017): 158–162, doi:10.1265/MSM.899490.

meres, and essentially become immortal. So, following the wisdom of the Dao, it is best to take the middle path. Maintain a balance of healthy exertion and restorative practices, minimize psychological stress, and maximize the nutrients in your food.

Unfortunately, the majority of us live in disequilibrium. We work too long and sleep too little. We sit for hours without moving. We eat processed takeout food while running from one activity to the next. We find it difficult to maintain healthful behaviors such as cardiovascular exercise, meditation, tai chi, qigong, or yoga. Living out of harmony with the Dao has taken its toll, individually and collectively. Over the past several decades, startling changes have occurred in the general health of the American population with respect to lifestyle-induced chronic conditions, such as heart disease, diabetes, digestive disorders, Alzheimer's disease, chronic pain, and cancer. Chronic conditions are defined as diseases that are noninfectious, last a long time, do not resolve by themselves, and are seldom completely cured. The majority of these illnesses are caused by unhealthy lifestyle choices: poor diet, lack of exercise, and smoking.

About 70 percent of all deaths in the United States are attributable to chronic conditions. More than 130 million Americans suffer from at least one chronic disease. That's about half of all adults in the United States, many of whom have considerable limitations in all aspects of their lives. Aside from individual suffering, chronic disease exacts a toll on the nation. The cost of caring for all these people with chronic conditions utilizes 86 percent of the country's health-care expenditures.[4] Predictions from various sources indicate that the prevalence of these diseases will only increase in the coming decades.[5]

---

4. Centers for Disease Control and Prevention, "Chronic Disease Overview," https://www.cdc.gov/chronicdisease/overview/index.htm.

5. American Heart Association, "Forecasting the Future of Cardiovascular Disease in the United States," January 24, 2011, http://circ.ahajournals.org/content/early/2011 /01/24/CIR.0b013e31820a55f5.abstract; American Diabetes Association, James P. Boyle, "Projection of Diabetes Burden through 2050," November 2001, http://care.diabetes journals.org/content/24/11/1936.full; World Health Organization, "Preventing

But the real shock is what our current lifestyle choices are doing to our children. In the 1960s, less than 2 percent of American children and adolescents had any chronic illnesses. By 2004, that number had almost quadrupled, to 8 percent. That increase is scary enough, but the next data point is even more disturbing. In 2007, more than 25 percent of our children and adolescents suffered from a chronic disease.[6] This is truly astounding. If you graphed out these data points, you would get an exponential curve. This means that in the not-too-distant future, if unchecked, *all* our children will suffer from one or more chronic illnesses such as diabetes, heart disease, hypertension, asthma, obesity, or cancer.

So, why is this happening, and what can we do about it? First, from a Western perspective, let's look at the biology of chronic disease. At first glance, there may not seem to be a link between all of the aforementioned chronic diseases. Certainly, diabetes, heart disease, hypertension, and obesity are often seen together. But what about the others? Chronic pain, arthritis, digestive disorders, Alzheimer's, asthma, depression? It may not be obvious, but all share a common thread. Disruption of cellular function on a molecular level can be caused by chronic inflammation, oxidative stress (the by-product of biochemical processes within the cell), and shortened telomeres.[7] Chronic inflammation leads to oxidative stress and telomere shortening. Soon, the damage is too great, and the cell cannot recover. At that point, the cell initiates a "self-destruct program" called apoptosis.

Inflammation in and of itself is not a bad thing. In fact, inflammation is a critical process in healing. It is the body's normal response to

Chronic Disease," http://www.who.int/chp/chronic_disease_report/presentation/en/index.html (accessed January 30, 2014).

6. National Institutes of Health, "Chronic Condition Self-Management in Children and Adolescents," December 11, 2013, http://grants.nih.gov/grants/guide/pa-files/PA-14-029.html.

7. Clara Correia-Melo, Graeme Hewitt, and Joao F. Passos, "Telomeres, Oxidative Stress and Inflammatory Factors: Partners in Cellular Senescence?" *Longevity and Healthspan* 3 (2014): 1, doi:10.1186/2046-2395-3-1.

acute injury or infection. If you scrape your knee or catch pneumonia, white cells within your blood release certain chemicals, called inflammatory markers. These markers tell your body to increase blood circulation to the affected area. Your knee, for instance, will start to look redder and feel warmer following the injury. These are signs that your immune system is responding correctly. The greater blood circulation will bring more nutrients and infection-fighting cells to the damaged part of your body.

If you could not mount a proper immune response, you would die. You would succumb to the first viral or bacterial infection that came along. However, it seems that something has gone awry on a very large scale. It has been discovered that constant low-grade inflammation contributes significantly to chronic disease because the immune system starts to attack normal tissue throughout the body.

This sort of inflammation, dubbed "meta-inflammation"[8] or "whole body inflammation,"[9] is not a response to acute injury or infection but, rather, is induced by our lifestyle habits. While it is true that environmental toxins can also cause inflammation, we can still reduce our risk for chronic disease by making better decisions. Our choices surrounding food, alcohol, cigarettes, exercise, sleep, and stress management heavily influence our immune systems. By continually making poor choices, we have overwhelmed our bodies. In computer parlance, there is a saying: "Garbage in, garbage out." From a Western perspective, chronic disease is the logical result of long-term input that promotes inflammation and tissue damage.

Eastern medicine looks at chronic illness in much the same way. As we discussed in the first chapter of this book, good health is regarded as a natural consequence of balanced living. Blood and qi flow easily through all the channels of the body. Essence, energy, and spirit are in

---

8. Wendy Kohatsu, MD, "The Anti-Inflammatory Diet," in *Integrative Medicine*, 3rd ed., ed. David Rakel, MD (Philadelphia: Saunders/Elsevier, 2012), 2297.

9. Andrew Weil, MD, "Reducing Whole Body Inflammation? - Ask Dr. Weil," https://www.drweil.com/diet-nutrition/anti-inflammatory-diet-pyramid/reducing -whole-body-inflammation/.

harmony. All this is primarily achieved through moderate diet, exercise, sleep, and meditative practices. While acupuncture and herbs figure prominently in Eastern medicine, adherence to a healthful regimen is the cornerstone of this healing system.

When your diet is poor, when you do not get enough sleep and exercise, or when you are under stress, your body becomes vulnerable, slightly weakened, and energetically unbalanced. From an Eastern viewpoint, diseases arise because of such imbalances. These disturbances can have an external or internal source and could involve not only the body but the mind and the spirit as well. The symptoms may be subtle, at least from the point of view of a Western practitioner who may not be trained to elicit or acknowledge these indicators of impending disease.

One of the strengths of Eastern medicine is the recognition that particular patterns of symptoms and signs may indicate imbalance. If left uncorrected, these energetic dysfunctions will lead to disturbances of qi and blood circulation and ultimately organ disharmony. In using the word "organ," we are referring to not only the anatomic structure of an organ, but also its physiology, its function, and its areas of influence throughout the body. In Eastern medicine, nothing exists in isolation. A disturbance in one channel or organ will affect all the others. This is an elegant explanation of the neurological, immune, and endocrine systems at work. After so many years of trying to reduce the human body to the smallest component, Western physicians are starting to return to the concept that the intricate interplay between larger systems determines a person's state of health.

Now, you are probably asking, "Can anything be done to reverse this epidemic of chronic illness?" What with all the chemicals in our water and air, all the unhealthy fats inserted into processed food, and all the stressors of modern life, good health seems like a lost cause. But you *can* take control of your own well-being. The World Health Organization (WHO) and Centers for Disease Control (CDC) have determined that simply by exercising more, eating better, and not smoking, 40 percent of cancers and 80 percent of heart disease and adult-onset diabetes could be prevented.[10]

Not so simple, you say? True, it can be difficult to initiate lifestyle changes. That is why chapter 5 of this book is devoted entirely to helping you overcome inertia and make better choices. But there is one thing you can start right now that will decrease chronic inflammation and make a huge difference to your overall health.

Eat More Plants

Even if eating more plants is the only change you make, your health will improve significantly. If you eat a healthy diet based on plants, you could decrease your chance of developing a chronic disease by at least 60 percent.[11] You do not need to become a vegetarian, but you need to make fruits and vegetables the mainstay of your diet. More and more Western biochemical research has determined why fruits and vegetables are essential for good health. Western doctors are returning to the wisdom of their forebears, like Hippocrates, who said, "Let food be your medicine and medicine be your food."

Of course, practitioners of Eastern medicine have never forgotten this basic tenet of healthy living. They have always stressed the importance of eating plants. Why can eating plants decrease your risk for chronic disease? Because the nutrients within plants act like medications that reduce inflammation. These compounds act on specific biochemical reactions in the body and have many beneficial effects. Aside from supplying high concentrations of vitamins and minerals, plant proteins, such as those in certain legumes, nuts, and seeds, are rich in healthy fats (omega-3 fatty acids) that have anti-inflammatory effects.

---

10. Kenneth Thorpe and Jonathan Lever, "Prevention: The Answer to Curbing Chronically High Health Care Costs (Guest Opinion)," May 24, 2011, http://www.kaiserhealthnews.org/Columns/2011/May/052411thorpelever.aspx.

11. Wendy Kohatsu, MD, "The Anti-Inflammatory Diet," in *Integrative Medicine*, 3rd ed., ed. David Rakel, MD (Philadelphia: Saunders/Elsevier, 2012), 2297.

Now that you know how a plant-based diet will reduce chronic inflammation, let's take a look at other dietary and lifestyle choices you can make to reduce inflammation and optimize your health.

Inflammation and Fat

Fat is crucial to your health. Every cell in your body needs fat. Fats are used to build cell membranes and cover your nerve cells. Fats play a role in the production and storage of energy, the transportation of oxygen, and the regulation of inflammation.

However, not all fats are created equal. While saturated fats, such as butter and coconut oil, should be used sparingly, and artificial fats, called trans-fats, should be avoided at all costs, monounsaturated and polyunsaturated fats have nutritional benefits. Healthful monounsaturated fats are found in such foods as olive oil, nuts, avocados, and sunflower oil. The fatty acids in polyunsaturated fats come in two types: omega-3 fatty acids (canola oil, flaxseed oil, walnuts, and fatty coldwater fish) and omega-6 fatty acids (corn, soybean, and safflower oil).

Both omega-3 and omega-6 fatty acids are essential fatty acids (EFA) that we cannot make ourselves. We need to get them from food sources. Whereas omega-3 fatty acids exert an anti-inflammatory effect, omega-6 fatty acids promote inflammation. Remember, inflammation is a natural component of the healing process. We can't do without it, or without omega-6 fatty acids. The problem is that the ratio of omega-6 to omega-3 fatty acids has changed drastically over time. A healthy ratio is considered to be about two to one (omega-6 to omega-3), but the standard American diet, high in processed foods, unhealthy fats, and sugar, creates a huge imbalance of as much as twenty-five to one. Elevated levels of omega-6 fatty acids have been associated with thicker blood that is prone to clotting. It also causes tightening and spasms of the arteries. Small wonder such a diet increases the risk of heart disease. Blood cannot flow freely through the body. Also, because both of these EFAs use the same enzyme and biochemical pathways, the more omega-6s we eat, the less omega-3s we process.[12] Because of this imbalance, we are not even getting the maximum benefit from the healthy fats that we do eat.

We can correct this disparity by choosing foods that are minimally processed and high in omega-3 fatty acids. While plants should make up the majority of the foods you eat every day, additional anti-inflammatory advantage can be obtained by consuming fatty, cold-water fish or eggs that have been fortified with omega-3 fatty acids. These recommendations are the basis of the "anti-inflammatory diet." Of course, there is no one diet that lays claim to this title. The Mediterranean and Okinawan diets are traditional ways of eating that emphasize whole, unprocessed foods, healthy fats like fish oil and olive oil, abundant fruits and vegetables, and minimal amounts of lean animal proteins and sweets. (For a more in-depth description of an anti-inflammatory diet and a worksheet to help you improve your food choices, please refer to appendix A.)

Inflammation and Sugar

For many years we have been urged to cut out the fat in our diet in an effort to decrease heart disease. Our supermarkets are overflowing with low-fat products, but heart disease and other chronic diseases are on the rise. It turns out the real culprit is sugar.

As a society, we eat excessive amounts of highly refined carbohydrates in the form of white sugar and white flour. These are metabolized too rapidly and cause abnormally high levels of glucose and insulin in the body. Our cells try to process all this extra glucose, but simply can't keep up. The mitochondria in our cells (the structure inside cells where energy is produced) get completely overwhelmed; they can't work fast enough. As a consequence, the majority of the glucose is incompletely

---

12. Wendy Kohatsu, MD, "The Anti-Inflammatory Diet," in *Integrative Medicine*, 3rd ed., ed. David Rakel, MD (Philadelphia: Saunders/Elsevier, 2012), 2301.

metabolized, which leads to the formation of molecules called free radicals. These molecules cause a lot of damage to the cells, particularly the cells that line the arteries, a condition known as oxidative stress. The immune system responds to this cell injury in the arteries, using cholesterol-laden plaques to essentially repair the damage. Persistently elevated blood sugar leads to chronic inflammation. It is the inflammation that renders the plaque more susceptible to rupture, causing a heart attack or stroke. Moreover, all this cellular damage slows down the normal metabolism, and so even more glucose is incompletely processed, causing a downward spiral of cell damage and inflammation. This sequence of events demonstrates the link between elevated blood glucose and cardiovascular disease.[13]

On the other hand, eating whole, unprocessed carbohydrates, like brown rice, bulgur wheat, and quinoa, slows down digestion and the release of glucose and insulin into the bloodstream. The mitochondria can completely process the glucose, and dangerous by-products are sharply reduced. The difference in the speed at which whole foods are digested is due to the increased amounts of fiber they contain: there is an inverse correlation between dietary fiber and oxidative stress with resulting inflammation. This means the more fiber you ingest, the less inflammation in your body. Fruits and vegetables are considered complex carbohydrates because they are essentially made of natural sugars: they are unprocessed and unrefined. They are beneficial for many reasons, not the least of which is the large amounts of fiber they contain.

As mentioned above, fruits, vegetables, and whole grains are the basis of an anti-inflammatory regimen. Not only will these foods supply large amounts of fiber, they also supply magnesium, zinc, B vitamins, vitamin E, and lignans, all of which help decrease inflammation.

---

13. Antonio Ceriello, MD, PhD, "Diabetic Complications: From Oxidative Stress to Inflammatory Cardiovascular Disorders," July 2011, http://www.medicographia .com/2011/07/diabetic-complications-from-oxidative-stress-to-inflammatory -cardiovascular-disorders/.

So, how can you tell which foods will give a consistent, even release of glucose and won't overload your mitochondria? Check their glycemic load. You may have already heard of the glycemic index, a measure of how quickly a food is digested into simple sugars within a specific time. The glycemic load is similar, but it gives more information.

The glycemic index uses a standardized amount of white bread as its reference point because white bread is metabolized so quickly and causes striking increases in blood sugar levels after it is eaten; it is assigned a value of 100. Research has been done that compares how the same amount of other foods affect blood sugar levels in the same amount of time. The glycemic index of a food is assigned a number between 1 and 100, based on how quickly it raises blood sugar values compared with white bread. For example, an apple has a low glycemic index value because it causes a lower rise in blood sugar levels compared with white bread in the same amount of time.

Glycemic load uses the glycemic index but goes a step further. It also takes into account the amount of carbohydrates that a food contains in a typical serving. When you compare foods, you find that those foods with a low glycemic index will also have a low glycemic load, but those with a high glycemic index may go either way once the carbohydrate content is considered. Foods that have rapidly digestible sugar but also a high water content will have a high glycemic index value but a low glycemic load. This is because there is relatively little sugar in an average serving of the food.[14] Watermelon is a good example.

Using either the glycemic index or glycemic load values is a good way to choose foods that will reduce your risk of chronic disease due to inflammation. Using the glycemic load also has additional benefits. Research has shown that diets based on low-glycemic-load foods are easier to sustain and result in decreased food cravings, spontaneously smaller portion sizes, and increased weight loss.[15] (For a list of the

---

14. Sarah K. Kahn, RD, MPH, PhD, "The Glycemic Index/Load," in *Integrative Medicine*, 3rd ed., ed. David Rakel, MD (Philadelphia: Saunders/Elsevier, 2012), 2287.
15. Ibid., 2288.

glycemic index and glycemic load of common foods, please refer to appendix B.)

Inflammation and Spices

Some Americans lack spices in their diets. Spices contain phytonutrients and other compounds that fight oxidation and inflammation,[16] the processes underlying most chronic disease (diabetes, heart disease, arthritis, digestive disease, autoimmune disease). Spices make food more attractive: it tastes good, smells good, and you feel good after a meal. Spices in food act as a mood enhancer, and spicy food stimulates the brain.[17] Spices that are particularly useful in decreasing inflammation are turmeric, ginger, cayenne, rosemary, oregano, cumin, garlic, cinnamon, cloves, and sage.

Inflammation and Obesity

At one time, fat cells were thought to be simply a storage site for excess calories. Actually, fat is metabolically active and is now considered to be the body's largest hormone-producing organ. Hormones produced by fat cells (adipose tissue) are called adipokines. One adipokine called adiponectin has anti-inflammatory effects, but the more fat a person carries, the lower the levels of adiponectin. This loss of the protective effect of adiponectin leads to a state of chronic inflammation.[18] It is thought that this is the common pathway for the development of other diseases such as diabetes, hypertension, and heart disease. In some respects, it is difficult to know which came first, obesity or inflammation.

---

16. Wendy Kohatsu, MD, and Scott Karpowicz, MD, "Antiinflammatory Diet," in *Integrative Medicine*, 4th ed., ed. David Rakel, MD (Philadelphia: Saunders/Elsevier, 2018), 877.

17. Dr. Aihan Kuhn, *True Brain Fitness* (New York: iUniverse, 2010).

18. Vivian C. Luft et al., "Chronic Inflammation Role in the Obesity-Diabetes Association: A Case-Cohort Study," *Diabetology and Metabolic Syndrome* 5 (2013): 31, doi:10.1186/1758-5996-5-31.

Inflammation and Alcohol

Excessive alcohol consumption can cause inflammation.[19] Many people don't realize the damage alcohol can do to the body and the brain. Chronic alcohol abuse can affect the brain and cause memory issues and dementia later in life.

In the short term, too much alcohol can inhibit the absorption of certain vitamins and minerals that can lead to problems with metabolism, the sleep cycle, and the musculoskeletal system. Aside from all the psychosocial problems that can arise, alcohol can also play a role in obesity and malnutrition.

Inflammation and Mind-Body Interventions

Mind-body interventions are techniques that can be used to activate the brain to change the body. These techniques include meditation, qigong, tai chi, yoga, hypnosis, and biofeedback. They can be used to decrease stress and pain by reducing chronic inflammation.

Here is how it works: when people are exposed to chronic stress in the form of psychological or physical pain, the "fight or flight" response is activated, and the body turns on proinflammatory genes via a factor called nuclear factor kappa B (NF-kB). The body is preparing to respond to injury. The substances that the proinflammatory genes produce are called cytokines. Cytokines can initiate inflammation. Under normal circumstances, the brain then activates neurotransmitters and hormones that decrease inflammation, but with long-term stress, the body becomes less sensitive to these anti-inflammatory signals. Chronic inflammation results.

High levels of NF-kB correlate with increased inflammation. By measuring levels of NF-kB in research subjects, a variety of studies have

---

19. H. Joe Wang, Samir Zakhari, and M. Katherine Jung, "Alcohol, Inflammation, and Gut-Liver-Brain Interactions in Tissue Damage and Disease Development," *World Journal of Gastroenterology* 16 (11): 1304–1313, doi:10.3748/wjg.v16. i11.1304.

shown that mind-body interactions decrease NF-kB levels and, therefore, inflammation.[20]

Inflammation and Exercise

For thousands of years, healers of all traditions have recommended exercise. It was, and still is, considered integral to a long and productive life. From an Eastern perspective, exercise improves the flow of blood and qi, nourishing all aspects of the body and mind. Acknowledging the association between regular exercise and good health, Western researchers have investigated why this is so.

Population-based studies have demonstrated the association between exercise and low levels of chronic inflammation.[21] This sort of study is like taking a snapshot of a group of people. An association between two conditions may exist, but the design of the study cannot show a definitive cause and effect. More recently, studies designed to show a cause and effect have been performed. One such study used four groups of moderately overweight or obese people and followed them over a twelve-week period.[22] One group performed aerobic exercise, one group performed resistance training, one group did both, and one group did no exercise at all. Blood samples that measured markers for inflammation were taken from all groups at the beginning and end of the study. The greatest decrease in inflammatory markers was seen in the group that did both aerobic and resistance exercises, followed by the resistance-training group, then the aerobic exercise group. No change was noted in

20. Ivana Buric et al., "What Is the Molecular Signature of Mind-Body Interventions? A Systematic Review of Gene Expression Changes Induced by Meditation and Related Practices," *Frontiers in Immunology* 8 (June 2017): article 670, doi:10.3389/fimmu.2017.00670.

21. K. M. Beavers, T. E. Brinkley, and B. J. Nicklas, "Effect of Exercise Training on Chronic Inflammation," *Clinica Chimica Acta* 411 (11-12): 785–793, doi:10.1016/j.cca.2010.02.069.

22. S.S. Ho et al., "Effects of Chronic Exercise Training on Inflammatory Markers in Australian Overweight and Obese Individuals in a Randomized Controlled Trial," *Inflammation* 36 (3): 625–632, doi:10.1007/s10753-012-9584-9.

the control group. This study demonstrated that exercise causes a decrease in inflammation within the body.

Knowing that exercise can reduce inflammation, it is easy to see how regular exercise can help prevent chronic disease. But that is not all that exercise does. Its beneficial aspects are numerous. Exercise enhances heart strength, efficient metabolism, all hormonal balances, immunity, and mental health.

As you read through this book, you will find more information and strategies that will help you start an exercise regime. If you are already an avid exerciser, congratulations! You are well on your way to vibrant health, free of the damaging effects of chronic inflammation.

Inflammation and Smoking

One would think that, in this day and age, smoking would have become a thing of the past. It should be unimaginable that anyone would ever smoke, given the insurmountable evidence of its dangers. Unlike eating, there is no necessity to smoke. In spite of the well-documented connection between smoking and disease, an estimated forty-three million adult Americans smoke. That doesn't even include children who smoke. It is estimated that about one in five high school students smokes.[23] Unfortunately, once someone has started smoking, it is incredibly difficult to quit. Smoking is addictive.

Most people understand that smoking is directly linked to lung cancer and respiratory illnesses, but fewer are aware of its connection to chronic illnesses like heart disease, stroke, diabetes, and even infertility.[24] The underlying mechanism of disease is the damage caused to

---

23. Centers for Disease Control and Prevention, "Chronic Disease at a Glance," http://www.cdc.gov/chronicdisease/resources/publications/aag/chronic.htm (accessed January 28, 2014).

24. US Department of Health and Human Services, "A Report of the Surgeon General: How Tobacco Smoke Causes Disease—The Biology and Behavioral Basis for Smoking—Attributable Disease Fact Sheet," http://www.surgeongeneral.gov/library /reports/tobaccosmoke/factsheet.html (accessed January 30, 2014).

the body by chemicals within cigarette smoke. Cancers are caused when these chemicals cause derangements in the DNA of the cells, the genetic code found in each cell of the body. Chronic degenerative diseases are caused by the constant inflammatory response that the immune system mounts to contend with persistent cell damage. This can affect any part of the body.

The good news is that if a smoker quits, the body will heal itself to a considerable extent. After the first smoke-free year, the risk for having a heart attack decreases significantly. After two to five years, the risk of having a stroke drops to roughly the same as a nonsmoker's. After five years, the risk for cancer of the mouth, throat, esophagus, and bladder are halved. Even the risk for dying of lung cancer decreases by 50 percent after ten smoke-free years.[25]

Looking at the changes in the inflammatory response, it has been shown that markers of chronic inflammation decrease to levels seen in nonsmokers by five years after a person has quit smoking.[26] It is never too late. Given a chance, your body will do its best to heal. That is its natural response. If smoking is a habit that you hope to modify, the advice and exercises in chapter 5 will help you achieve this extremely important goal.

Inflammation and Sleep

Americans tend to "burn the candle at both ends." Not only is our workweek longer than that of many other industrialized countries, but vacations are shorter. Also, Americans tend to stay awake late into the night, usually watching TV or surfing the internet. All this activity takes time away from sleep.

---

25. Ibid.

26. Arvind Bakhru and Thomas P. Erlinger, "Smoking Cessation and Cardiovascular Disease Risk Factors: Results from the Third National Health and Nutrition Examination Survey," *PLoS Medicine* 2 (6): e160, doi:10.1371/journal.pmed.0020160, PMCID: PMC1160573.

In 2013, the average number of hours we slept in the United States was six and a half hours per night. This is much less than the eight-hours-per-night average documented during the 1950s.[27] An hour and a half less each night doesn't sound like such a big deal, and it wouldn't be if it were just once and a while. The problem is the cumulative effect of getting too little sleep. According to the CDC, 30 percent of Americans get fewer than six hours of sleep each night.[28] For teenagers, it is even worse. They require nine hours of sleep every night, and many are consistently getting only five!

We clearly do not value our sleep. Many people do not realize how important sleep is to our neurological, endocrine (hormonal), and immune systems. Lack of sleep has been associated with chronic inflammation,[29] decreased immunity, and disrupted hormone secretions that affect not only our sleep/wake cycle but the way our bodies metabolize energy and heal. Chronic sleep disruption has even been designated as a risk factor for cancer. Adequate sleep is critical to brain processing and memory consolidation. During sleep, special channels in certain brain cells open to allow waste products and toxins to drain, thereby keeping the brain functioning well.[30] Inadequate sleep has been associated with the abnormal expression of over seven hundred genes.[31] This in turn can affect the way the body replenishes itself and, ultimately, lead to degenerative diseases.

---

27. Russell Foster, "Why Do We Sleep?" TED Talk, June 2013, http://www.ted.com/talks/russell_foster_why_do_we_sleep.html.

28. *Huffington Post*, "Sleep Deprivation Affects Genes," February 26, 2013, http://www.huffingtonpost.com/2013/02/26/sleep-deprivation-genes_n_2766341.html.

29. Janet M. Mullington, PhD, Norah S. Simpson, PhD, Hans K. Meier-Ewert, MD, and Monida Haack, PhD, "Sleep Loss and Inflammation," *Best Practice and Research: Clinical Endocrinology and Metabolism* 24 (5): 775–784, doi:10.1016/j.beem.2010.08.014.

30. Norman Doidge, MD, *The Brain's Way of Healing* (New York: Penguin, 2015), 112.

31. *Huffington Post*, "Sleep Deprivation Affects Genes," February 26, 2013, http://www.huffingtonpost.com/2013/02/26/sleep-deprivation-genes_n_2766341.html.

A great deal of research has been done in recent years that demonstrates that genes that control normal sleeping patterns are linked to genes responsible for normal mental health. Sleep disturbances coexist with many serious psychiatric diseases, such as bipolar disorder, depression, anxiety disorder, and schizophrenia. In fact, abnormal sleep patterns usually precede mental illness in predisposed individuals. Researchers have used this fact to help such patients. By treating the sleep disturbances, manifestations of psychiatric illness can be decreased by as much as 50 percent.[32] Sleep disruption can be used as an early warning system that something in the body is amiss.

For centuries upon centuries, the Chinese have been concerned about sleep quality as it relates to overall health. At last, Western science is starting to catch up. Research has shown that good-quality, restorative sleep is associated with better health and increased concentration, attention to detail, creativity, and social and decision-making skills. Poor-quality, non-restorative sleep is related to failing health, impulsiveness, stress, anger, mood swings, substance abuse, poor memory, and motor vehicle accidents (more than one hundred thousand per year in the United States). To quote the British neuroscientist Russell Foster, "Sleep is not an indulgence."[33]

True, everyone stays up late to party or has difficulty sleeping once in a while, but caution is advised. Recurring and severe lack of restorative sleep, known as insomnia, is easier to prevent than to treat. It is better to recognize inadequate sleep habits and correct them before it is too late and chronic insomnia sets in. Such interventions may also minimize the effects of certain mental illnesses. To decrease the chance that you will ever need treatment for insomnia, incorporate the following recommendations into your daily routine:[34]

---

32. Russell Foster, "Why Do We Sleep?" TED Talk, June 2013, http://www.ted.com/talks/russell_foster_why_do_we_sleep.html.

33. Ibid.

34. Rubin Naiman, PhD, "Insomnia," in *Integrative Medicine*, 3rd ed., ed. David Rakel, MD (Philadelphia: Saunders/Elsevier, 2012), 231.

- Exercise regularly, performing both cardiovascular exercise and "meditative" exercises such as tai chi, qigong, or yoga that will promote relaxation.
- Minimize the use of stimulants (like caffeine) and sedatives (like alcohol or sleeping pills).
- Keep a regular sleep/wake schedule by waking up at about the same time every day, getting exposure to morning light, dimming your lights an hour or two before bed, and going to bed at around the same time each night.
- Use your bedroom only for sleep or sexual activity, and banish all electronic devices such as televisions, computers, and cell phones.
- Sleep in complete darkness.
- Pay attention to recurring dreams or nightmares. They may be trying to tell you something important!
- If you cannot sleep after lying in bed for fifteen minutes, get up and do something restful, like meditate or take a warm bath; then try again. Do not lie awake in bed watching the clock!
- Find healthy, constructive ways to manage stress, such as exercise, socializing with family and friends, meditation, qigong, and tai chi.
- Consult your physician if you have persistent difficulty sleeping.

Reducing your risk for chronic, debilitating disease is well within your capability. Even if you are already affected by a chronic condition, you can take control of your lifestyle choices and make a positive impact on your health. Taking steps to reduce the levels of chronic inflammation in your body will improve your metabolism and cardiovascular system. This is a modern way of saying what the ancient Chinese have always advocated; that is, follow the middle road and moderate your habits to improve the flow of blood and qi. Either way you say it, you will achieve good health.

Now you have an understanding of the cause of chronic disease from both the Western and Eastern perspective. Given current projections, you are also aware of what is at stake—not only your own personal health, but the physical and fiscal health of the country. It is not an understatement to say that if chronic illness is not prevented, the world economy is in jeopardy.

Reversing the epidemic of lifestyle-induced disease is a complicated matter. Taking personal responsibility for maintaining your health is an excellent start, but, as the saying goes, "No man is an island." You are part of an enormously complex health-care system. Understanding how that system emerged and functions is essential. In chapters 3 and 4, we discuss the origins and current state of health care in America and how to integrate Eastern medicine into that structure to ensure your own well-being. Armed with that knowledge, the remainder of this book will help you devise your own step-by-step path toward optimal health.

CHAPTER 3

Our Current Health-Care System

The American Paradox

You may have heard of the "French paradox," the fact that the French seem to be able to drink alcohol and eat rich foods yet still maintain good health. Well, America has its own paradox: we spend vast amounts of money on health care, but we are in terribly poor health as a society. In fact, for all the money that has been spent, our actual health is among the worst of all industrialized countries.

Let's look at just a few categories:

- Avoidable deaths
- Life expectancy
- Infant mortality

Avoidable Deaths

Avoidable deaths (known as avoidable mortality) is a measure of how well a nation's health system can cure a condition that is, in fact, curable. The United States came in last among nineteen developed nations on this parameter, largely due to lack of universal access to care. If you are under seventy-five with a curable illness and you live in America, you are two times more likely to die from that disease than if you lived in France, Japan, or Spain.[1]

---

1. T. R. Reid, *The Healing of America: A Global Quest for Better, Cheaper, and Fairer Health Care* (London: Penguin, 2010), 28.

So, if you have a curable ailment, you are more likely to die if you live in the US. What if you have a chronic, incurable condition, like asthma or diabetes? Would you fare better because of all the newer treatments and medications that are available here? Sadly, no. In a study that looked at how patients with chronic conditions fared in nine industrialized countries, asthmatics died sooner in the US than in any other country aside from Great Britain. Diabetics in America ranked last in terms of life expectancy within this group.[2]

Life Expectancy

With respect to life expectancy, the United States lags behind the majority of European countries as well as industrialized Asian ones. One could argue that this result is a misrepresentation, since many more Americans die in the prime of life due to car accidents and violent crimes than do young Europeans, for example. So, to take a more even-handed approach, we can look at a marker that medical researchers call "healthy life expectancy at age sixty." This does not mean how long a person will live after the age of sixty, but rather how many more years a person will be healthy after the age of sixty. As such, this statistic is a good indicator of how well a nation's health-care system takes care of its populace. Unfortunately, in this 2006 survey, the United States was tied for last among twenty-three other industrialized countries.[3] Moreover, in the United States, for the first time in many decades, this number is decreasing. That means that children born today will enjoy fewer years of good health in their senior years than will their parents.

Infant Deaths

Speaking of children, let's look at another parameter of a nation's well-being: the infant mortality rate. This is a statistic that tells you how many newborn babies die within one year of birth. The infant mortal-

---

2. Ibid., 32.
3. Ibid., 33.

ity rate is twice as high in America than other developed countries, in spite of incredible advances in neonatal intensive care. That means that despite greater proportions of specialized pediatricians (neonatologists) and intensive-care beds that are available in the US, a baby is still more likely to die before his first birthday in the States than in other wealthy countries.

One might argue that American neonatologists are more willing to attempt to save babies that are born on the cusp of viability, at earlier and earlier gestational ages. This could skew the statistics, as these newborns are more likely to die than those born full term, but if you compare the infant mortality rate in America with countries that have similar practice patterns, like Canada, the US still fares poorly.

This disparity is due in no small part to the lack of free prenatal and neonatal care in America. Every other industrialized country has a well-organized national system to ensure that all pregnant women receive comprehensive prenatal care. Disability and maternity leaves in other countries are far more generous than in the US. In other comparably wealthy nations there are no financial barriers to babies receiving adequate medical care. Taken together, these factors contribute to fewer premature births, lower infant mortality rates, and better overall infant health than is seen in America.[4]

The Costs of Health Care

So, it seems that the old saying, "You get what you pay for," does not apply in the United States. There is no denying that America's system is the most expensive in the world. In 2007, $2.3 trillion were spent on health care; that was 16 percent (or one-sixth) of the gross national product for the year. In 2009, those numbers rose to $2.5 trillion, and 17.6 percent of the GNP.[5] The United States spends at least 50 percent more per person on medical expenses than any other nation. Yet

---

4. Ibid., 28.

5. Kaiser Family Foundation, http:www.kff.org (accessed July 27, 2012).

Americans suffer with ill health to an alarming degree.[6] For all the money that is spent on medical care, you might expect to see better outcomes, but no other country on earth spends so much and gets so little in return.

This fact is glaringly obvious in a report published by the World Health Organization in 2000. The WHO created a formula to determine the "overall achievement" of the health systems of 191 countries. This group comprised industrialized and nonindustrialized nations. The study looked at the level of health of the population, distribution of health care, and fairness of financial contributions. The results were notable for the fact that the United States ranked thirty-seventh in a field of 191. Not bad, you say? Well, consider that, in 2000, America spent almost $5,000 per person, greater than 50 percent more than most other wealthy nations, and yet had the lowest healthy life expectancy of that subgroup at sixty-nine years of age. In 2009, we spent more than $8,000 per person, yet over the past decade the rates of diabetes, cancer, and heart disease are higher than ever before. How can this be?

That question has no simple answer. There are many, many reasons why our medical system is as expensive and inefficient as it is today, including

- patchwork health-care distribution
- lack of universal access to care
- medical waste
- the medical-industrial complex
- increasing reliance on expensive technologies and medications
- disproportionate number of specialists
- inability to prevent chronic lifestyle-driven illnesses

Let's look at each of these issues separately to try to understand the intricacies of this complicated problem.

---

6. Andrew Weil, MD, *You Can't Afford to Get Sick: Your Guide to Optimum Health and Health Care* (New York: Plume, 2009), 53.

Patchwork Health-Care Distribution

By the end of the 1990s, health-maintenance organizations (HMOs) and managed-care companies accounted for the majority of private health-care distribution systems. Although these "for-profit" entities were initially able to bring some costs down, such as doctors' fees, they had no control over the prices charged by drug companies and medical-device manufacturers. Some countries have single-payer systems, meaning the government pays for the people's health care, funded by taxes collected from individuals and corporations. Because the government is the single payer, it is able to set the price these companies will receive for their products. Some aspects of the American system have this advantage, including Medicare, Medicaid, and the Department of Defense, which oversees care given to military personnel. HMOs lack this advantage. The drug companies and medical-device manufacturers take advantage of this lack of control by charging more for their products, leaving the insurance companies to absorb the costs. Actual drug costs tripled during the 1990s, even though the cost to the patient decreased. This led the insurance companies to increase their premiums further. In fact, since 1999, premiums for employer-sponsored health insurance have increased four times faster, on average, than workers' earnings, and almost five times faster than inflation.[7]

Lack of Universal Access to Care

Let's leave the moral implications of limited access to health care aside for the moment. From a very practical point of view, millions of Americans are uninsured and can only access medical care through hospitals when in dire emergencies. These people are often working and earn too much money to be considered eligible for federal or state medical assistance programs. Of the fifty million Americans without insurance

---

7. Kaiser Family Foundation, http:www.kff.org (accessed July 27, 2012); Andrew Weil, MD, *You Can't Afford to Get Sick: Your Guide to Optimum Health and Health Care* (New York: Plume, 2009), 23.

in 2009, 77 percent were from working families, and 69 percent were from low-income working families with average annual wages of 200 percent of the poverty level. (In 2009, the poverty level for a family of four was $22,050 per year.) Such individuals often cannot afford private health insurance when their employer does not offer this benefit. Surveys show that the uninsured are six times more likely to postpone medical care because of cost and seek attention only when they are very sick. Because they are unable to see a doctor at the beginning of an illness, when intervention is usually simpler and less expensive, they may find themselves in emergency departments with conditions that are more serious than when they began. The patient, the hospital, or the government must absorb the higher costs of these visits. Had these people been able to see a doctor when their conditions were simpler to treat, they would have been spared needless suffering, and the medical system would have been spared needless expense.

Medical Waste

Western medical practices, particularly in the hospital-based acute-care setting, generate a phenomenal amount of waste. Medical waste is an extremely complex entity. It is not composed only of the usual garbage that any large business would produce, such as paper, cardboard, and plastic. Medical waste also includes chemicals, radioactive isotopes, pharmaceuticals, and potentially infectious biological substances like blood. Though considerable care and expense is taken in processing medical waste, it still has a long-standing economic and environmental impact.

It is difficult to pinpoint how much medical waste is produced annually, the exact cost required to process it, or the effect on the ecosystem, but here are some estimates tabulated by various agencies over the past decade:

- Hospitals use approximately 836 trillion BTUs of energy annually, making them the second most energy-intensive buildings in the country. This energy usage contributes significantly to greenhouse gas emissions. The health-care sector is estimated to be responsible for 8 percent of all greenhouse gas emissions in the United States.[8]

- Hospitals are significant water consumers, using between 40 and 350 gallons per capita per day.[9]

- In a 2010 survey of 114 hospitals that participate in the environmentally minded network called Practice Greenhealth, the average amount of waste generated was 33.8 pounds per day per staffed bed.[10] That's 12,337 pounds per staffed bed per year. That is double the estimate of 6,600 pounds per year that was put forward in the early 1990s. In 2012, the American Hospital Association estimated there are about 940,000 staffed beds in the country.[11] This works out to roughly 5.8 billion tons of waste annually.

- Of this 5.8 billion tons of waste, approximately 15 percent is considered hazardous. That equals about 870 million tons of biohazardous waste that must be specially processed. The cost differential is substantial. The estimates for processing ordinary waste and medical waste are $25 per ton and $480 per ton, respectively.[12]

- At an estimated cost of processing of $93 per ton (given that each ton contains 15 percent biohazardous waste), the expense of processing 5.8 billion tons of hospital waste is about $540 billion annually.

- Biohazardous medical waste can include hazardous gases, toxic metals, and pharmaceuticals. In spite of improving methods of disposal, these noxious substances can work their way into our air,

8. J. W. Chung and D. O. Meltzer, "Estimate of the Carbon Footprint of the US Health Care Sector," *JAMA* 302 (18): 1970.

9. Energystar, http://www.energystar.gov/index.cfm?c=health care.ashe_sept_oct_2005 (accessed July 20, 2012).

10. Practice Greenhealth, http://practicegreenhealth.org/topics/waste (accessed July 29, 2012).

11. American Hospital Association, http://www.aha.org/research/rc/stat-studies/fast-facts.shtml (accessed July 29, 2012).

12. American Recycler, http://www.americanrecycler.com/0810/357medical.shtml (accessed July 29, 2012).

soil, and watersheds. Environmental pollutants have been shown to be at least partially responsible for the increasing rates of cancers, asthma, and neurological diseases found in our communities.[13]

In recent years, American health-care facilities have made great strides in waste management. These improvements have followed the same "reduce, reuse, and recycle" philosophy that is gaining momentum throughout the country. Many hospitals have made efforts to use renewable energy, recycle cardboard and paper, and implement safer methods of disposing of hazardous waste. In the operating room, clean but unused disposable surgical instruments are being sent to developing countries that may lack basic supplies. There is also a movement afoot to make available more reusable, sterilizable medical equipment, as was done in the past. Where prepackaged disposable procedure kits are used, there is often a large number of wasted instruments, so medical personnel are requesting that the manufacturers streamline these products, eliminating excessive wrapping and increasing the likelihood that all the instruments in the kit will be utilized.

A great deal can be done to diminish the size of the carbon footprint of America's health-care sector, but the single greatest factor in controlling the environmental impact of Western medicine technology is a decrease in its use. There will always be a need for the emergency room and operating room in every community. Unfortunately, accidents and catastrophes will happen. However, for every patient who avoids a coronary artery stent, a gastric bypass, or hospital stay for the complications of diabetes, there will be a reduction in the amount of medical waste produced. Only by adhering to the tenets of preventive medicine, which includes Eastern medicine, will we see a truly significant decline in the trash and pollutants generated in the acute-care setting.

---

13. Practice Greenhealth, http://practicegreenhealth.org/topics/waste (accessed July 29, 2012).

The Medical-Industrial Complex

The topic of the business of medicine is very complicated. In fact, whole books have been written about how the medical industry has affected our health. It is important to understand how the business of medicine affects us on a daily basis.

More than thirty years ago, Dr. Arnold Relman, editor of *The New England Journal of Medicine* (1977–1991), warned of the dangers of an "investor-owned" health-care system. He likened the change in the way medical care was administered to President Dwight D. Eisenhower's astute observation of the shift in national defense. President Eisenhower warned that the commercialization of the country's military support organizations would lead to war for the sake of profit. The comparison is truly striking. Relman contends that as the medical industry strives to increase its profit, it will do so at the expense of efficient and effective care.[14]

Take the treatment of type 2 diabetes as an example. This condition can be greatly ameliorated, if not completely controlled, by adequate exercise and a nutritious diet. There were twenty-six million type 2 diabetics in the United States in 2010—over 8 percent of the population, or roughly one type 2 diabetic for every twelve Americans. In addition, there were an estimated seventy-nine million prediabetics. These numbers have increased greatly over the last decade, and it is projected that, by 2050, one out of every three Americans will be diabetic.[15]

All these diabetics would be taking blood-sugar-lowering medications and using devices to check their glucose levels several times a day. While the diabetes epidemic represents a huge challenge to the health-care system, it will be a tremendous boon to the manufacturers of these drugs and devices. In 2010, the actual medical cost incurred by type 2 diabetics in the United States was $116 billion. If even half of these

---

14. Andrew Weil, MD, *You Can't Afford to Get Sick: Your Guide to Optimum Health and Health Care* (New York: Plume, 2009), 69.

15. Centers for Disease Control and Prevention, October 22, 2010, www.cdc.gov /media/pressrel/2010/r101022.html.

people were able to control their disease through lifestyle changes alone, corporate profits would plummet. A similar loss of income would be seen if people with elevated blood pressure were able to use fewer medications, as is often the case when they lose weight and exercise.

A healthy population benefits America as a society by decreasing federal expenditures on medical costs and increasing individual productivity; however, a robust citizenry benefits medical corporations not at all. Is it any wonder that these companies spend so much time and money to promote the use of their expensive medications and devices? These products treat the symptoms and consequences of these conditions but do not treat the cause. There are effective and inexpensive modalities that would. These include moderate exercise and a healthful diet of whole foods, as advocated by many Western physicians and practitioners of Eastern medicine.

Of course, the purpose of these businesses is to make money. They often pay lip service to lifestyle changes, but many of them would suffer considerable financial losses if we all paid attention to those recommendations.

So whose businesses are we talking about? The large pharmaceutical companies, recently known as Big Pharma, the medical-device manufacturers, and all their lobbyists on a statewide and federal level.

Now, no one is suggesting that drug and device companies be abolished. In many cases, certain medications and medical instruments are nothing short of lifesaving. Examples include antibiotics for severe infections, insulin for type 1 diabetes, and mechanical heart valves for those whose own heart valves have ceased to function. But for all these items that could be deemed essential, there are as many, or more, that have proven to be more expensive, less effective, and even dangerous when compared to treatment with nutritious food, adequate exercise, and supplementary low-tech strategies. Let's look at a few examples.

The New England Journal of Medicine, in 2002, published a study funded by the marketers of a certain cardiac defibrillator. This device is implanted in the hearts of patients who have life-threatening irregular heartbeats. If the heart suddenly stops beating, the defibrillator will automatically deliver a dose of electricity to restart the heart. Implanted defibrillators have saved many lives of such patients; however, in this study, the defibrillators were used in people who had suffered a heart attack, but did not have a life-threatening heartbeat. The results demonstrated that there was a 31 percent drop in heart attacks in the following twenty months. At first glance, this looks impressive, but as not all of these heart attacks were fatal, the cost of saving a single life was a staggering $1.5 million.[16]

Moreover, this study did not cite other studies that had demonstrated less expensive methods to prevent considerably more deaths in such patients. In 1999, *Circulation* published a study demonstrating that moderate exercise decreased the risk of death by 63 percent. Compare this result to the defibrillator study above, which decreased the risk of heart attack by 31 percent. Also, moderate exercise produced an increase in exercise capacity and quality of life. Another study in 2000 in the *Archives of Internal Medicine* showed that smoking cessation had a significant effect in decreasing the risk of death. Compared with defibrillators, smoking cessation had 1.5 to two times as much benefit as the defibrillators, at a fraction of the cost.[17]

Let's take a look at diabetes again. It has been estimated that 91 percent of the risk of developing type 2 diabetes can be attributed to poor diet, excessive weight gain, lack of exercise, and smoking. If you are overweight, you are 7.5 times more likely to become afflicted with type 2 diabetes than if your weight is in the healthy range. If you are obese, that risk rises to twenty times.[18] All these risk factors are modifiable, but for the vast majority of Americans, medications to lower blood sugar are the first line in treatment. Now there is a trend toward put-

---

16. John Abramson, MD, *Overdosed America: The Broken Promise of American Medicine* (New York: Harper Collins, 2004), 100.

17. Ibid., 101.

18. Ibid., 230.

ting all these diabetics on cholesterol-lowering medications, known as statins, since diabetics are more likely to have heart disease—another way in which pharmaceutical companies stand to make a large profit. Medications are given greater emphasis than lifestyle changes in spite of various studies that show that diet and exercise are superior to drugs in the treatment of type 2 diabetes. It has been shown that walking for at least two hours per week has decreased the death rate in diabetics by 39 percent. That works out to saving four lives per 250 patients each year. Compare this with the use of cholesterol-lowering medications in diabetics, which saves only one life per 250 patients each year.[19]

A Swedish study demonstrated that very modest weight loss (approximately five pounds) maintained over five years lowered the death rate by 83 percent in diabetic men compared with a control group of diabetic men who didn't lose weight. When compared to the addition of statins, the modest five-pound weight loss had a five-times-greater benefit. Another study placed diabetics into an intensive weight-loss program for twelve weeks. The amount of money spent on prescription drugs and supplies for these diabetics decreased by two-thirds after the program, and by one year after the study, these participants were spending only half of what they had previously on medications and devices.[20]

As a last example, let's look at cardiac procedures. These procedures are commonly done in the United States after someone has had a heart attack. A cardiac catheterization is a way of seeing the arteries of the heart and determining the extent to which atherosclerosis, also called plaque, has blocked them. The other procedure is a balloon angioplasty, which uses a balloon placed inside the blocked arteries to open up the plaques from the pressure of the balloon. Both of these procedures are invasive and not without risk.

Cardiac catheterizations and balloon angioplasties are five times and 7.5 times more common in the United States than in Canada, but the

---

19. Ibid., 231.
20. Ibid.

survival rate at one year out from the initial heart attack is no different. Americans are spending a lot more money for the same results. Comparing Americans to Americans, a study was done looking at the same procedures in New York and Texas. In Texas, 50 percent more of these procedures were performed than in New York, but the outcomes were worse. In Texas, after these procedures, the death rate was 15 percent higher, the rate of chronic chest pain (angina) was 40 percent higher, and 60 percent of people were unable to perform the activities of daily living they could have done previously.[21]

Clearly, more drugs or procedures are not the answer to creating a healthy population, but it is the answer to those who stand to make a profit from them. This includes not only the drug companies and medical instrument manufacturers, but also the hospitals that offer these procedures and the doctors who perform them. The medical-industrial complex has managed to gain an enormous amount of influence over our health. These corporations stand to lose a lot of money if people take matters into their own hands and if doctors are given the resources required to implement programs and motivate patients to become healthier. It is in the best interest of these corporations to forward the notion that expensive technologies are superior to low-tech grassroots strategies, and they advance their agenda in many ways.

In his excellent book *Overdosed America*, Dr. John Abramson sheds light on the methods used by medical corporations to undermine our health.

- The undue influence that medical corporations have exerted on the Food and Drug Administration in recent years
- The trend toward the commercialization of medical research, such that physicians are unable to trust the results
- The increasing pressure that industry lobbyists place on politicians at all levels of government
- Direct-to-consumer marketing

---

21. Ibid., 171.

- Persuading doctors to confine their treatment recommendations to the newest, most expensive technologies available (which these companies produce, of course)

Let's examine these factors individually.

The Food and Drug Administration (FDA)

The FDA is a regulatory body whose function is to determine the safety and efficacy of drugs and devices before these treatments reach the American public. Initially, the FDA was a completely independent body, composed of physicians, scientists, pharmacists, and other health-care professionals. These individuals are experts in their field and, by law, are not supposed to have any financial ties to the companies whose products they will be evaluating.

Unfortunately, because of a decrease in government funding and pressure to review and approve more drugs and devices in less time with fewer personnel, the FDA has grown to depend on funding from medical corporations and has begun to employ experts who do have financial interests in the companies in question.[22]

In a *USA Today* report in 2000, it was noted that, between 1998 and 2000, over eight hundred waivers regarding financial ties had been given to the FDA in order to hire enough expert personnel to fill the vast numbers of requests for product review. As such, 54 percent of the experts on the advisory committee had "a direct financial interest in the drug or topic they were asked to evaluate."[23] To use a popular aphorism, it is like leaving the fox to guard the chicken coop. It is extremely unlikely that such individuals will be completely impartial and unbiased in their assessment of the benefactor's product.

As a consequence, some drugs and devices have received FDA approval even though they show no advantage over those products already available. Some of these newer medications and instruments also have

---

22. Ibid., 89.
23. Ibid.

dangerous side effects. The number of drugs that had to be withdrawn from the market after receiving approval through the accelerated review process quadrupled following its implementation in the mid-1990s.[24]

Abramson cites the approval of Rezulin as an egregious example. Rezulin was a medication used in the treatment of type 2 diabetes and was the first diabetes drug to undergo the abbreviated review process. Dr. John Gueriguian, a FDA medical officer, raised concerns regarding liver toxicity in research subjects. He recommended that Rezulin should not receive FDA approval. Subsequently, Dr. Gueriguian was removed from the case following complaints from Rezulin's manufacturer, Warner-Lambert. When the final report was sent to the advisory committee, the council that would approve the drug, Dr. Gueriguian's concerns were not in the document.[25]

Rezulin did receive FDA approval in February 1997. It was sold worldwide, but by December 1997 was withdrawn in the United Kingdom because of reports of liver toxicity. The even more astonishing fact is that Rezulin continued to be sold in the United States for another twenty-eight months until it was finally withdrawn in March 2000 because of numerous complications associated with the drug. There were 391 deaths and at least four hundred cases of liver failure. During this time, Warner-Lambert realized $2 billion in profit.

Commercialization of Medical Research

Prior to 1970, the vast majority of medical research was performed in academic settings, specifically universities or medical institutions; the funding source was governmental. Between 1970 and 1990, government support decreased, and by 1990, fully two-thirds of research grant requests were not funded. At this point, medical corporations increased their financial support to allow research to continue. By 1994, a great deal of medical research was commercially funded, but four-fifths of these studies took place in academic institutions, where strict adherence

---

24. Ibid., 86.
25. Ibid., 87.

to widely accepted standards of ethical experimental design and data analysis was still the norm. If a product was found to be ineffective or dangerous, then this would be declared in the results of the study.

Apparently, this arrangement did not suit the medical industry, as they increasingly took their research funding to commercial companies whose sole purpose was to run medical trials for those who paid them. By the year 2000, only one-third of clinical studies were performed in academic settings. The remaining two-thirds were implemented by companies that performed medical research for profit.

This would all be well and good if these commercial medical research companies were impartial, but unfortunately, this is not the case. Numerous studies have shown that a product is more likely to have a favorable result if the study is funded by the product's manufacturer. In fact, the likelihood is at least four times greater that the sponsor's product will be found to be safe and efficacious when the study is commercially funded than if it is performed by an organization that has no financial interest in the outcome.[26]

Also, by employing for-profit medical research businesses, drug and device companies have more control of the experimental data. In many instances, these hired researchers were not allowed to see all the data from the very experiments they were performing.[27] In other cases, studies have been cut short, or designs revised, to facilitate the manufacturer's desired outcome. These practices have become so pervasive that in September 2001, the editors of some of the world's most distinguished medical journals warned against the commercialization of medical research. Together, the editors of the *Journal of the American Medical Association*, the *New England Journal of Medicine*, the *Lancet*, and the *Annals of Internal Medicine* stated that "studies repeatedly document the bias in medically sponsored research."[28] Unfortunately, even such prestigious journals are unable to completely rid themselves of

---

26. Ibid., 97.
27. Ibid., 105.
28. Ibid., 96.

these sorts of research papers. There is great financial pressure from the medical industry, whose advertisements, to a large degree, fund these journals. If medical journals rejected all questionable studies, then they may cease to be fiscally viable. As Dr. Abramson so aptly stated, "The medical journals seem powerless to control the scientific integrity of their own pages."[29]

Lobbyists

Lobbyists are people who try to influence government officials to vote on legislation in a manner that would favor the lobbyists' interests. Lobbyists can come from a variety of sources. They can be volunteers or they can be professional lobbyists, hired by an organization to promote a particular agenda. Medical-device and pharmaceutical companies spend a lot of money every year to attempt to sway legislators to vote in favor of laws that would benefit these corporations.

Between 1990 and 2000, the pharmaceutical industry spent $177 million on governmental lobbying. Of this, $20 million was spent on campaign contributions and $65 million on political advertising.[30] These numbers keep increasing. Comparing amounts spent on lobbying from 2008 to 2009, there was an overall increase.[31] Let's look at just a few of these companies.

- The industry trade group Pharmaceutical Research and Manufacturers of America (PhRMA) spent $26 million in 2009, an increase of 29 percent.
- Pfizer Inc. spent almost $22 million in 2009, an increase of 80 percent.
- Amgen Inc. spent $12.4 million in 2009, an increase of nearly 23 percent.

While lobbying is certainly legal, there have been some ethical concerns regarding the "revolving door" of lobbyists who begin their

---

29. Ibid., 97.

30. Ibid., 90.

31. Open Secrets, January 2010, www.opensecrets.org/news/2010/01/new -lobbying-reports-show-big.html.

careers working for the government and then change jobs to work as lobbyists. The Obama administration tried to limit this trend by establishing stricter guidelines in this area. Even so, you can be sure that lobbying for the benefit of corporate interests will continue.

Direct-to-Consumer Marketing

All those ads on TV and the internet that suggest that you "talk to your doctor" about one medication or another is part of a strategy pharmaceutical companies call "direct-to-consumer (DTC) marketing." The name really says it all. These companies do not consider you as individuals or even as patients, but only as consumers of a commercial product. Prior to 1985, DTC marketing was not even legal in the United States. In fact, aside from New Zealand, the United States is the only other country in the world that allows drug companies to directly canvas "consumers." These corporations must abide by certain regulations, but in 1997, these became even more lenient.

Direct-to-consumer marketing is a way of circumventing the usual doctor-patient interaction when it comes to treatment plans. Normally, if the patient does indeed need medication, the doctor prescribes an appropriate drug, but also tries to use a cost-effective brand. If there is no compelling medical reason to use a more expensive alternative, it only makes sense to be economical when prescribing medications. Doctors do understand that, somehow, these drugs have to be paid for. When patients request newer and therefore more expensive medications, they may not be willing to listen to reasons to use other ones that are tried and true. Doctors may also feel pressured to grant the request, for no other reason than the desire to please the patient. Some doctors also do not wish to appear confrontational by pointing out that some newer medications may not be as clinically effective or cost-effective as older drugs or lifestyle changes.

Drug companies are very keen on this marketing approach because, if the physician does prescribe their product, their sales will obviously increase. Pharmaceutical companies know that the patient will pay only a small portion of the cost of a drug through a co-pay because, if they have insurance, that health insurance company is obligated to pick up the remainder of the tab. Because of the way the American health-care system is structured, health insurance companies have little or no control over the cost of pharmaceuticals and devices. In countries where there is a single-payer system, the government sets the price it will pay for these products. In such countries, the profits reaped by medical corporations are not as astronomical as they are in the United States.

Persuading Doctors

Just as medical corporations try to influence patients with direct-to-consumer marketing, they also try to influence doctors. Over the years, stricter guidelines have been established regarding the sorts of interactions that drug or device company representatives can have with medical personnel. In the past, considerable amounts of money were spent on commercial support for continuing medical-education functions. These functions often involved elaborate venues, expensive food, free medical texts, and some office supplies. Although this behavior has decreased over the years, it still occurs, and it has been shown that the greater the interaction between doctors and drug representatives, the greater the likelihood that those doctors will prescribe the products in question.[32]

Another way in which drug companies try to influence doctors is by monitoring their prescribing habits. Pharmacies sell this information to the drug companies, which then send drug representatives to doctors' offices to inquire as to why the doctor is not using the company's product. In 2007, Vermont tried to ban the sale of this information unless the doctor consented to it. This state law was overturned by the US Supreme Court in 2011, stating that the commercial transfer of prescribing practice information was protected by free-speech laws.[33] That means

32. John Abramson, MD, *Overdosed America: The Broken Promise of American Medicine* (New York: Harper Collins, 2004), 126.

33. Michelle M. Mello and Noah A. Messing, *"Restrictions on the Use of Prescribing Data for Drug Promotion,"* September 29, 2011, *N Engl J Med* 2011; 365:1248–1254, DOI: 10.1056/NEJMhle1107678.

this data can be bought and sold without a doctor's consent, unless that doctor specifically opts out of the process by registering their intent through the American Medical Association.[34]

Perhaps the worst outcome of the association between doctors and the medical industry is the pervasive view that only the newest, most advanced technology can be effective in combating illness. The marketing techniques of these companies, their manipulation of research results, and their influence on the Food and Drug Administration have insidious and far-reaching effects. The goal of medical corporations is to make money, to turn a profit for shareholders. We should not expect the medical-industrial complex to have our best interests at heart. However, we should expect that from ourselves and our doctors. Our doctors ought to be able to help us determine which mode of therapy will be most beneficial to us, as individuals and as a society.

Increasing Reliance on Expensive Technologies and Medications

The commercialization of the practice of medicine is driving up the cost of health care in America. While many drugs, devices, and procedures available are truly miraculous, study after study has shown that commonsense approaches increase quality and length of life to a greater degree than do expensive technologies. These commonsense approaches are not new: regular exercise, not smoking, getting enough sleep, stress management, and an unprocessed diet that is rich in beneficial fats. These modifications increase healthy life expectancy by many, many years by preventing the onset of chronic illnesses. The Chinese have advocated similar strategies for thousands of years: inexpensive lifestyle changes are the cornerstone of Eastern medicine.

Such simple actions cost very little, yet they would save the country billions and billions of dollars. First, millions of Americans would not

---

34. American Medical Association, www.ama-assn.org/go/pdrp (accessed July 27, 2012).

suffer from chronic diseases such as diabetes or heart disease; money would be saved by decreasing the incidence of these conditions. Second, with each intervention, such as cardiac catheterization or arterial bypass surgery, complications inevitably occur. Without these millions of interventions, even more money would be saved by avoiding the necessity of treating the complications. It is estimated that complications from adverse drug events alone cost $200 billion each year. That is not including the cost of complications from medical procedures.

So, who is responsible for our lack of common sense? We all are.

From the pharmaceutical and medical-device companies to the FDA, from processed-food manufacturers to physicians, from medical schools, political lobbyists, and health insurance companies down to each of us as individuals, we are all responsible for this predicament.

Of course, each of these entities is responsible in its own way, for its own reasons. Various factions promote our reliance on expensive technology predominantly because of one of two things: either the desire to reap financial rewards or the misguided notion that high-tech treatment yields superior long-term results.

In addition to the belief that more technology delivers better results, doctors overuse expensive diagnostic technologies for three other reasons. The first is the fear of litigation. In a 1993 survey, 60 percent of physicians who responded admitted to ordering more diagnostic tests than truly needed because they worried about being sued. In 2008, the American Medical Association conducted a survey and found that that number had greatly increased, with 93 percent of responding physicians admitting they have practiced this sort of defensive medicine. Even if they are virtually certain of the diagnosis based on the patient's history of the presenting illness and their physical exam, there is a strong tendency for doctors to order extra tests to rule out uncommon diseases. They do this to avoid being sued for missing a rare diagnosis. It is unusual these days for a physician to treat a patient based on the clinical evaluation alone. Before, if a patient did not improve as expected, then the doctor would go on to order tests. Many physicians are unwilling to use this approach, as it carries a small risk of failing to diagnose an eso-teric disease; however, the cost of these extra tests is estimated at almost $230 billion annually.[35]

The second reason that doctors order excessive tests has to do with the way they are trained. It has been said that more than 90 percent of a diagnosis will be discerned from the patient's history and physical exam. The emphasis that has been placed on these skills has diminished as availability of diagnostic modalities has increased. In places and time periods in which these advanced technologies were in short supply, phy-sicians had to rely almost completely on their diagnostic acumen.

The third reason that physicians order unnecessary tests is the strong urge to "do something." It is very difficult for doctors, particularly those in the United States, to allow enough time for a condition to either declare itself or resolve. There is an undeniable tendency to order more tests, pre-scribe more drugs, or perform more procedures than may be necessary. Sometimes this behavior is driven by the patients, and their expectation that they will walk out of their doctor's office with "something" in hand, either a prescription or test order. The recent trend of drug and medical-device companies directing their advertising toward the public has reinforced this behavior. It becomes very hard for American doctors and patients alike to accept that "watching and waiting" is not "doing noth-ing." It is allowing the body to undergo the normal process of healing. In these circumstances, the physician can best serve the patient by making recommendations that support this natural process. As we shall see, it may not be in the patient's best interest to take more pills or undergo an expensive battery of tests and procedures. It will, however, cer-tainly drive up the cost of health care.

Disproportionate Number of Specialists

Another way medical education in America drives up the cost of care is in the number of specialists that are trained in relation to the number

---

35. Pacific Research Institute, "Health Policy Prescriptions," October 2009, www .pacificresearch.org/health-care/.

of family practitioners. Over the years, there has been a steady increase in the number of specialists and subspecialists and a corresponding decrease in the number of family physicians.

In his book *Overdosed America*, Dr. John Abramson states that "comparisons both within the U.S. and between countries show that access to comprehensive, family-centered, primary care service is the distinguishing characteristic of health-care systems that are both effective at producing good health and efficient at controlling costs." Generally, in America, the higher proportion of specialists has led to increased costs to the system. The greater the number of specialists, the greater the cost. This is because specialists' fees are higher, and specialists are more inclined to performed procedures. After all, that is what they are trained to do. The problem is that, in many areas, more procedures may not improve health outcomes.

It has been determined that an efficient proportion of primary care doctors to specialists should be 50 percent, but in 2002, it was found that only 21 percent of physicians in the United States were primary care doctors. That number fell by more than 25 percent between 2002 and 2007.[36] The *Wall Street Journal* reported in April of 2010 that, in spite of a push to boost the numbers of family physicians, there could be a shortage of 150,000 primary care doctors by 2025.[37]

There are several reasons for this disparity. During a doctor's training there is a perception, whether true or not, that there is more prestige attached to being a specialist than a family doctor. From a financial perspective, specialists command higher salaries and fees than do their generalist colleagues.

Finally, to a young doctor embarking on specialist training, there can be some comfort in having a narrower field of study, with the hope that they can learn everything about one area of study. Family doctors

---

36. John Abramson, MD, *Overdosed America: The Broken Promise of American Medicine* (New York: Harper Collins, 2004), 82.

37. Suzanne Sataline and Shirley S. Wang, "Medical Schools Can't Keep Up," *Wall Street Journal*, April 12, 2010, http://online.wsj.com/article/SB100014240527023 04506904575180331528424238.html.

have a more daunting task: they are expected to know almost everything about everything! They must have a firm foundation in all aspects of medicine—cardiology, dermatology, gynecology, pediatrics, psychiatry, and infectious disease, to name but a few. They must also get their patients to lose weight, quit smoking, and wear their seat belts. For all this, in spite of their equally staggering debt from medical school, family doctors get paid, on average, only half of a specialist's salary. Is it any wonder that fewer new doctors are choosing to become family physicians?

While the disproportionately high number of specialists is understandable, it is driving up the cost of our medical care. The more troubling issue, as we have seen, is that the quality of our health as a nation is considerably lower than in other countries where specialists are fewer and where the majority of the population is treated by primary care doctors.

Inability to Prevent Chronic Lifestyle-Driven Illnesses

The cost of treating chronic illnesses in the United States accounts for 75 percent of the health-care budget. For the year 2009, when $2.5 trillion was spent on medical care overall, almost $1.9 trillion was allocated to the treatment of chronic diseases such as type 2 diabetes, heart disease, hypertension, stroke, and cancer; 70 percent of all deaths in America are attributable to these chronic illnesses. That is an incredible waste of lives and money when you consider that a large percentage of these conditions could have been prevented by a healthier diet, more exercise, and smoking cessation. True, everyone must die someday, but wouldn't it be so much better to die in one's sleep from old age than suffer a debilitating stroke or a painful death from cancer?

Not all chronic illnesses can be prevented by optimizing one's health, but study after study has shown that the benefits of exercise, proper diet, adequate sleep, and smoking cessation outweigh any benefit conferred by medical procedures or pharmaceuticals. Here is a summary of a few of these studies:

- The benefit of exercise is two times greater than the benefit of an implantable cardiac defibrillator in preventing death in patients with an irregular heartbeat.[38]
- The benefit of smoking cessation is 1.5 to two times greater than a cardiac defibrillator in preventing death in patients with an irregular heartbeat.[39]
- The benefit of the Mediterranean diet (less red meat, healthier fats such as olive oil and nuts, lots of fruits and vegetables) is three times greater than statin drugs in reducing heart disease in patients that already have that diagnosis.[40]
- The benefit of exercise is almost five times greater than that of medication in mild depression.[41]
- The benefit of exercise produces a risk reduction of 40 to 50 percent for colon cancer and 30 to 40 percent for breast cancer.[42]
- The risk of getting one of the following cancers increases if you are obese: ovarian (by 95 percent), colon (by 90 percent), breast (by 66 percent), leukemia (by 61 percent).[43]

These statistics are only a tiny fraction of those published that have demonstrated the vast benefits of a healthy lifestyle compared with the benefits of expensive technologies. So why, with so much evidence, is it so difficult for our society to properly address the growing epidemic of preventable disease by using simple and economical strategies? Once again, there is no straightforward answer.

---

38. John Abramson, MD, *Overdosed America: The Broken Promise of American Medicine* (New York: Harper Collins, 2004), 100.

39. Ibid.

40. M. de Longeril et al., "Mediterranean Diet, Traditional Risk Factors, and the Rate of Cardiovascular Complications after Myocardial Infarction: Final Report of the Lyon Diet Heart Study," *Circulation* 99 (6): 779.

41. John Abramson, MD, *Overdosed America: The Broken Promise of American Medicine* (New York: Harper Collins, 2004), 233.

42. Ibid., 234.

43. Ibid., 235.

As individuals, we must be willing to take the time and make the effort that such lifestyle changes require. However, being human, we are always looking for the effortless way out of a situation. It takes commitment to change lifelong habits, even when we know those habits can hurt us. Drug and medical-device companies are happy to let you think that the only and easiest solution to your problem is whatever they have to sell.

As a society, we have not prioritized the allocation of resources toward maintaining our own good health. On both business and governmental levels, it seems we are more willing to spend money on disease treatment than prevention. The CDC budgets only a small proportion for preventive medicine. Doctors are paid more, by all types of insurers, to treat illness than to prevent it in the first place.

Slowly, there does seem to be a paradigm shift occurring. Medical schools are increasing the percentage of the curriculum spent on nutrition, exercise physiology, stress reduction, and disease prevention. However, once these new doctors graduate, they find they are not appropriately compensated for helping their patients make meaningful lifestyle changes. In spite of these economic realities, physicians must continue to emphasize that prevention is safer, more efficient, and more cost-effective than the reactionary, high-tech approach of "modern" medicine.

In the next chapter we examine how, with the help of Eastern medicine, our health-care system can evolve to meet the challenges that we face in the twenty-first century.

CHAPTER 4

East Meets West

How to Get the Most Out of Your Health-Care System

The Importance of East-West Integration

It is clear that the current health-care system in the United States does not completely meet the needs of the people. It is also clear that this system is not going away, medically, economically, or politically. From a medical point of view, few would want to do without the fabulous life-saving technologies that biomedicine has discovered, such as antibiotics and surgery. Economically and politically, the country is deeply divided over the best way to offer medical care to the public. For better or worse, corporate-driven for-profit biomedicine is here to stay for the foreseeable future. The larger question for every individual is, how do we maintain optimal health within the structure that is available?

From this first question, many more come to mind: Is biomedicine alone the best system to manage chronic disease, lifestyle-related illnesses, or musculoskeletal ailments not amenable to surgery? Is biomedicine effective for chronic pain without masking it with addicting medications? Does biomedicine go to adequate lengths to prevent these conditions in the first place? Many would answer these questions with a resounding "No!"

So, how to fill in the gaps, to take advantage of the modalities at which biomedicine excels but supplement in the areas in which it struggles? Eastern medicine and those systems related to it certainly fit the bill and are uniquely suited to provide individualized therapies for both acute and chronic conditions. Many practitioners of Eastern medicine would agree that, in Western societies, the dovetailing of these two systems could offer effective treatment for almost every ailment.

For those unfamiliar with the benefits of Eastern medicine, other questions arise:

- What is Eastern medicine used for?
- Has Eastern medicine been researched?
- How effective is Eastern medicine?
- Could good results just be placebo effect?
- Is Eastern medicine safe?
- Why should we consider the integration of Eastern and Western medicine?
- Are Western physicians willing to incorporate Eastern modalities?
- How should I approach my doctor about using Eastern medicine?
- How should these two systems be used together?

We discuss all these issues in the coming pages. By the end of this chapter, the utility of integrating Eastern and Western medicine will be apparent.

What Is Eastern Medicine Used For?

When people think of Eastern medicine, they most commonly think of acupuncture. When they think of acupuncture, they instantly think of back pain. It is true that back pain is the first ailment for which Western countries accepted Eastern solutions. However, there is a vast array of different conditions for which all components of Eastern medicine can be used.

As we have already discussed, Eastern medicine is composed of various strands: acupuncture, herbal formulas, bodywork, tai chi, qigong, dietary therapy, exercise, and meditation. Any or all of these practices can be used to improve many chronic and some acute conditions. For certain life-threatening acute conditions, Western medicine would still be the modality of choice. If you had a shattered leg from a car accident, you'd want an orthopedic surgeon. If you had an overwhelming bacterial infection, you'd want intravenous antibiotics. If you were a woman in labor with a baby who was too big to be born naturally, you'd want a cesarean section. In our Western society, we all too often forget that the "natural" consequence of certain conditions is severe disability or death. In these situations, Western medicine shines, saving the lives of people who would normally die in another time or place where these techniques were not available.

But no system is perfect. What Western medicine lacks is the capacity to effectively treat many chronic illnesses. This is where Eastern medicine makes its greatest contribution. Many people are surprised to learn that Eastern medicine can be used for such diverse conditions as cardiac arrhythmias, digestive complaints, insomnia, gynecologic problems, infertility, and asthma. (A much more extensive list from the World Health Organization can be seen in the table in the subsection below that discusses treatment effectiveness.)

Has Eastern Medicine Been Researched?

If you were to go to your computer and use a common medical search engine such as PubMed to look for research articles on Eastern or Oriental medicine, you would find thousands. By searching the subject "East Asian medicine," you would be presented with over ten thousand papers. If you looked specifically for articles about acupuncture, more than seventeen thousand would appear.

It is one thing to say that research has been done, but it is important to know a little about how studies were designed and what questions they were set up to answer. These two questions are crucial, regardless of the modality being tested. It could be the latest drug for diabetes, the newest surgical technique, or a therapy as ancient as acupuncture. The question being posed and the study design are key to yielding meaningful results that can be applied to the individual patient.

Research itself is a relatively new concept. In Western medicine, up until around the Second World War, the effectiveness of a certain treatment was measured by the improvement of the patient. During that time, the validity of a therapy was based on the accumulated outcomes of its use. Over time, with repeated successes, practitioners incorporated an intervention into their usual practice. Those therapies that did not benefit the majority of patients were discarded. This is the manner in which Eastern medicine has developed over the millennia. It is a very practical way of looking at the utility of a treatment. The bottom line was this: Did the patient improve or not?

Just before the Second World War, researchers studied the effects of certain agricultural fertilizers on the growth of two groups of plants. One group was treated with the active substance and one group was not. The untreated group was designated the "control" group. So began the era of controlled trials.[1]

Then the idea of randomly assigning participants (human or otherwise) to either the clinical or control group gave rise to the randomized controlled trial, commonly referred to as an RCT. Randomized controlled trials were further refined by "treating" the control group with a placebo. In essence, the control group was managed in exactly the same way as the study group, except the control group was not given the active substance that was being tested. At the end of the trial, differences between the groups had to be sufficiently large to show that the active substance or treatment was having an effect. This is referred to as being statistically significant. It was no longer enough to say that a patient or group of patients improved after an intervention; now the improvement in the study group was required to be greater than the improvement seen in the placebo control group. As we shall see, this methodology has several problems, particularly with respect to Eastern medicine and acupuncture.

Randomized controlled trials are designed to answer a specific question: that is, does the treatment/drug/intervention being tested cause the observed effect? This sort of study design is said to be "explana-

1. Claudia W. Witt et al., "Efficacy, Effectiveness and Efficiency," in *Integrating East Asian Medicine into Contemporary Health Care*, ed. Volker Scheid and Hugh MacPherson (Edinburgh: Churchill Livingston/Elsevier, 2012), 190.

tory," and it looks at the efficacy of a treatment.[2] It is best suited to the sort of biochemical experiments seen in drug trials. This represents a simple cause-and-effect relationship between the intervention and the outcome. The expectation is that as long as all other factors remain unchanged, the same cause will always result in the same effect. RCTs are designed to test interventions on a homogeneous population in order to decrease variability between the treatment and placebo group and also within the groups themselves. Statistically significant results yield a great degree of predictability, and those results translate easily into clinical practice guidelines.

Unfortunately, the real world is somewhat more complicated. It has frequently been found that, in spite of excellent results during research trials, certain drugs or interventions do not give the same degree of benefit when applied to the general population. Within the general population there is a wider range of differences among patients. These differences can cover a multitude of areas, all of which can affect the treatment response. Some factors include age, gender, comorbidities (additional illnesses aside from the one being treated), compliance with the treatment regimen, socioeconomic status, family situation, and societal influences and expectations. Additionally, the practitioner who is administering the intervention can also influence the outcome. Here again, the factors are numerous and include level of training, innate skill, and the relationship that the practitioner has with the patient.

For the reasons stated above, there has recently been a keen interest in the biomedical community to adjust study designs, taking these complexities into account. In these instances, the study is not designed to determine whether a certain treatment causes a certain effect. In this sort of study, the treatment and control groups are still randomized. The initial structuring of the study is not that much different: it is the question that has changed. The new question posed is this: Does this intervention do what it is intended to do under real-world conditions, without regard for the exact mechanism of action? These sorts of studies are

2. Ibid., 191.

called "pragmatic" and are concerned only with effectiveness, not causality. In other words, did the patient get better or not?[3]

This is not to say that one type of study is better than the other. It is only meant to point out that you really need to know what question you are asking before you design a study. For a while now, biomedical researchers and medical anthropologists have been determining ways to investigate more complex biological systems that fall outside the realm of straight-ahead cause-and-effect reactions. This is similar to the way that the study of physics has shifted from investigating the linear world of Newtonian physics to the vastly more complicated universe of quantum physics.

Eastern medicine certainly falls into the category of a complex system. Many components and variables determine whether or not a treatment is successful, and this presents the greatest obstacle to researching the efficacy of Eastern medicine. On the other hand, the effectiveness of Eastern medicine has been demonstrated, both through clinical research and in everyday use.

How Effective Is Eastern Medicine?

In 2012, the World Health Organization updated its list of those conditions for which acupuncture was deemed useful. In this report, the evidence for acupuncture's utility was taken only from clinical trials that were formally published in peer-reviewed journals. These studies were required to have an adequate number of patients to observe an effect, in either randomized controlled trials or nonrandomized controlled trials. This means that in the randomized trials, patients were assigned at random to either the acupuncture group or the control group. In the control group, the patients received either conventional Western therapy or sham acupuncture. Sham acupuncture is a type of "pretend" acupuncture that will be explained in greater detail shortly. In the nonrandomized trials, those patients who received acupuncture were compared with

---

3. Ibid., 191.

similar groups of patients who did not, but none of the patients was randomly assigned into their groups.

Acupuncture was deemed useful to varying degrees in different clinical situations for an extensive list of ailments. The WHO divides the results into four groups:

- conditions for which acupuncture is definitely effective
- conditions for which there is a therapeutic benefit but more research is suggested
- conditions for which there is only some benefit but conventional therapies are problematic
- conditions for which acupuncture may be tried provided the practitioner has modern medical knowledge and means of monitoring the patient.

The majority of the studies reviewed for this report showed that acupuncture was beneficial.[4] Although many of the studies had a small number of participants (less than 100 people), most were randomized controlled trials. It may seem incredible that so many different conditions can be helped by acupuncture, but in our experience, the vast majority of patients will receive some benefit from treatment. As previously mentioned, the way in which acupuncture research is conducted is still evolving, and many studies stipulate that further research is needed.

The diseases or disorders for which acupuncture therapy has been tested in controlled clinical trials reported in the recent literature can be classified into four categories.

1. Diseases, symptoms, or conditions for which acupuncture has been proved through controlled trials to be an effective treatment:

   postoperative pain, renal colic, rheumatoid arthritis, sciatica, sprain, stroke, tennis elbow

---

4. World Health Organization, "Acupuncture: Review and Analysis of Reports on Controlled Clinical Trials," 2002, 23–26.

2. Diseases, symptoms, or conditions for which the therapeutic effect of acupuncture has been shown but for which further proof is needed:

abdominal pain (in acute gastroenteritis or due to gastrointestinal spasm); acne vulgaris; alcohol dependence and detoxification; Bell's palsy; bronchial asthma; cancer pain; cardiac neurosis; chole-cystitis, chronic, with acute exacerbation; cholelithiasis; competition stress syndrome; craniocerebral injury, closed; diabetes mellitus, non-insulin-dependent; earache; epidemic hemorrhagic fever; epistaxis, simple (without generalized or local disease); eye pain due to subconjunctival injection; female infertility; facial spasm; female urethral syndrome; fibromyalgia and fasciitis; gastro-kinetic disturbance; gouty arthritis; hepatitis B virus carrier status; herpes zoster (human [alpha] herpes virus 3); hyperlipemia; hypo-ovarianism; insomnia; labor pain; lactation deficiency; male sexual dysfunction; Ménière's disease; neuralgia, post-herpetic; neuro-dermatitis; obesity; opium, cocaine, and heroin dependence; osteo-arthritis; pain due to endoscopic examination; pain in thromboan-giitis obliterans; polycystic ovary syndrome (Stein-Leventhal syndrome); postextubation laryngospasm in children; postoperative convalescence; premenstrual syndrome; prostatitis, chronic; pruritus; radicular and pseudoradicular pain syndrome; Raynaud syndrome, primary; recurrent lower urinary-tract infection; reflex sympa-thetic dystrophy; retention of urine; schizophrenia; sialism; drug-induced Sjögren's syndrome; sore throat (including tonsillitis); spine pain; stiff neck; temporomandibular joint dysfunction; Tietze syn-drome; tobacco dependence; Tourette syndrome; ulcerative colitis; chronic urolithiasis; vascular dementia; whooping cough (pertussis)

3. Diseases, symptoms, or conditions for which there are only individual controlled trials reporting some therapeutic effects, but for which acupuncture is worth trying because treatment by conventional and other therapies is difficult:

chloasma, choroidopathy, central serous color blindness, deafness, hypophrenia, irritable colon syndrome, neuropathic bladder in spinal cord injury, pulmonary heart disease, chronic small airway obstruction

4. Diseases, symptoms, or conditions for which acupuncture may be tried provided the practitioner has special modern medical knowledge and adequate monitoring equipment:

breathlessness in chronic obstructive pulmonary disease; coma; convulsions in infants; coronary heart disease (angina pectoris); diarrhea in infants and young children; encephalitis, viral, in children; paralysis (progressive bulbar and pseudobulbar)

Even though this list of treatable conditions is extensive, it potentially underestimates the number of conditions for which acupuncture and, by extension, Eastern medicine can be effective, because of flaws in study design. For example, in the case of morning sickness in pregnancy, some studies show that acupuncture was as good as or better than standard medical treatment and certainly better than no treatment. Other studies were set up to compare women who received acupuncture against women who received sham acupuncture. Sham acupuncture has been variously described as needling prescribed points superficially, needling non-acupuncture points, needling points that have not traditionally been used for the condition being treated, or using retractable needles to simulate the experience of true acupuncture without the actual insertion.

In numerous studies, sham acupuncture has been shown to be as effective as true acupuncture. Those that doubt the usefulness of acupuncture interpret this as placebo effect; however, there are other plausible explanations. First, when using shallow needling, alternate points, or retractable needles, the acupuncture points are still being stimulated and are clearly having an effect. Second, with respect to the use of non-acupuncture points, this method either disregards or has no knowledge of the different schools of thought within Eastern medicine that employ the use of nonstandard points to achieve a clinical response. From an

Eastern perspective, nonstandard points are actually collateral points that communicate with the principal meridians in the same way that small blood vessels (capillaries) connect with larger arteries and veins in the circulation of blood.

To draw an analogy to Western medicine, if one could bypass the larger veins traditionally used for intravenous administration of drugs and somehow inject a medication into the tiniest capillary or even directly into a cell, one would see an effect. In the day-to-day practice of Western medicine, a similar method is actually used. For example, anticancer drugs can be injected into the abdominal cavity, not intravenously, and are absorbed by the body to fight cancer. A nonstandard method of administration still allows the treatment to have a positive effect.

From a Western perspective, the changes that result from sham acupuncture can also be explained. Recall that when any part of the body is stimulated, the pressure exerted on the collagen in our connective tissue creates a microcurrent of electricity. This microcurrent causes biochemical and neurological changes to occur, even if the effect is not as potent as when true acupuncture points are used. This explains why in some studies sham acupuncture can be better than no treatment and almost as effective as "real" acupuncture.

Could Good Results Just Be Placebo Effect?

The placebo effect has been seen in medical practice for centuries. The word "placebo" comes from the Latin, meaning "to please." The idea was that a doctor would give a patient a pill or treatment that was inert. If a pill, it contained no active substance. If a treatment or surgery, it engendered no actual intentional repair of any structure. In spite of this, a large number of patients actually improved or were cured. Historically, placebos have been used to encourage the patient's expectation that they would recover. From a research standpoint, placebos are used in an effort to ensure that the experience that both the study group and control group undergo is as close to the same as possible, to isolate the one active substance or intervention that is creating a change in the patient's condition. Introducing a placebo group into a randomized controlled trial is a common occurrence, but as we have seen, sometimes placebos confuse rather than clarify the results.

Even when a study involves a simple cause-and-effect response, such as testing a new drug, it is impossible to separate the human reactions of the participants, both patients and researchers. Medical anthropologists, such as Claridge and Helman, have pointed out for some time that there is a "total effect" of a drug or intervention that goes beyond the actual biochemical or physiologic nature of the treatment. The components that make up the total effect include the characteristics of the drug or treatment itself (even down to the color of the pill), the characteristics of the patient (age, gender, genetics, education, experience, personality, expectations), the characteristics of the researcher (personality, age, gender, attitude, professional status), and the setting in which the study is taking place.[5]

None of the above attributes can be removed from the clinical trial, and all of these characteristics are present within the study and placebo groups. This may explain, in part, why some patients who receive the active substance experience a negative clinical response and some within the placebo group improve.

So, does this mean that the positive clinical results experienced by placebo group patients are a figment of their imaginations? No. In many studies, the improvements seen in the placebo group can be objectively identified. These changes are not just qualitative, meaning the patient describes a state of improved health. The differences can also be defined quantitatively, such as findings of lower blood pressure and lower cholesterol levels, and the decreased use of painkillers.

How can these changes be occurring? There is a great deal of interest in the physiologic effects of the placebo. Around the world, researchers

5. Elisabeth Hsu, "Treatment Evaluation: An Anthropologist's Approach," in *Integrating East Asian Medicine into Contemporary Health Care*, ed. Volker Scheid and Hugh MacPherson (Edinburgh: Churchill Livingston/Elsevier, 2012), 234.

are documenting changes that occur in the immune system, the brain, the spinal cord, and the biochemical balance of the body in response to a placebo.

In many of these studies, the patient is not told that they are receiving a placebo. For many, this presents an ethical dilemma in the use of placebos in general practice. Interestingly, at Harvard's Program for Placebo Studies, Kaptchuk and others created a randomized controlled trial to look at the feasibility of using placebos without deceiving the patient.[6] All the patients had irritable bowel syndrome (IBS); they were randomized either to the open-label placebo group or the nontreatment control. Both groups received the same amount of time, counseling, and attention. Both groups were asked not to change any aspect of their usual routines for the duration of the study, such as starting a new diet or exercise program. Both groups had stable disease. The difference came at the end of the first interview, when the patients found out to which group they were assigned. The open-label group was told the pills they would take were "placebos, made of an inert substance, like sugar pills, that have been shown in clinical studies to produce significant improvement in IBS symptoms through mind-body self-healing processes."

The truly fascinating outcome of Kaptchuk's study was that even though patients knew they were taking placebos, their IBS symptoms improved more than those of the control group, which did not receive any pills. The statistically significant changes in the control group included decreased symptom severity and increased symptom relief. There was also a trend toward improved quality-of-life scores at the end of the study period for those taking placebos. Remember that these patients knew there was no medication of any sort in their pills. Still, they felt better and had scientifically measurable improvements in their IBS symptoms. This demonstrates that the power of the mind to heal the body is astonishing. Eastern medicine has always recognized that fact

6. T. J. Kaptchuk et al., "Placebos without Deception: A Randomized Controlled Trial in Irritable Bowel Syndrome," *PLoS ONE* 5 (12): e15591, doi:10.1371/journal.pone.0015591.

and uses it to full advantage by incorporating meditation, qigong, and tai chi into patient care.

Is Eastern Medicine Safe?

Any medical intervention can have unintended consequences, but generally speaking, Eastern medicine is safe if its procedures—such as acupuncture, *tui na* (therapeutic Chinese massage), diagnostics, and herbal prescriptions—are performed by well-trained practitioners.

Acupuncture is only one component of Eastern medicine. Herbal formulas are used frequently and are very effective for many conditions. These formulations can be used alone or in conjunction with acupuncture and other therapeutic modalities such as *tui na*, qigong, and dietary changes. Herbs, if properly prescribed and taken correctly, are safe to use. However, one must keep in mind that herbs must be prepared and administered with the same caution as any Western medication. Some people think that because herbs are "natural," they cannot be harmful, but this is not the case. Over thousands of years, the Chinese and other East Asian practitioners have determined the best ways to harvest, prepare, and combine herbs to create formulas that are effective and safe. Prescription errors, patient-compliance problems, and faulty manufacturing can cause serious side effects.

This is why it is important to be seen by a credentialed Eastern practitioner before purchasing any herbal remedies. It is imperative that the correct diagnosis be ascertained before a formula can be prescribed. Buying a remedy at your local health-food store or off the internet based on self-diagnosis could lead to incorrect treatment. Also, a provider who is properly trained in Eastern medicine can recommend reputable patent formulas or give you a custom blend of quality herbs from their own pharmacy. These practitioners are aware of the federal guidelines that apply to herbal supplements and should only recommend products from trustworthy companies.

Though herbs have pharmacologic actions, in the United States, they are not considered to be drugs. The regulation of herbs falls under the

Dietary Supplement Health and Education Act (DSHEA, 1994).[7] The DSHEA is an amendment to the Food, Drug, and Cosmetic Act, wherein herbs are classified as food—specifically, as a dietary supplement. This is in contradistinction to some other countries, like Australia, New Zealand, and China, where herbs are considered to be drugs and subject to the same regulations as pharmaceuticals.

In the United States, the guidelines governing the manufacturing and sale of herbs are not as stringent as those applied to drugs. Still, these regulations specify the rules that must be followed in the dietary supplement Current Good Manufacturing Practices (cGMPS).[8] These rules, set up to ensure quality and product safety, involve federal or state inspection of all aspects of manufacturing, including

- buildings and grounds
- air and water purification systems
- handling and processing of raw materials
- product-manufacturing processes
- operation and cleaning of equipment
- training of employees
- quality-control testing

Some manufacturers of both loose Chinese herbs and prepared formulas follow stricter guidelines and handle herbs as drugs, not food. These companies use only raw materials that are pure enough to be designated "medicinal grade." This means ensuring that the herbs are correctly identified and contain a sufficient amount of the active ingredient of the herb in each sample. It also means that no Western drug is added to the formula, as was done in decades past. The finished product is then tested for microbes (bacteria, yeast, and mold), toxic herbs, pesticides, and heavy metal content. The thresholds for acceptable levels

---

7. US Food and Drug Administration, "Dietary Supplements," http://www.fda.gov/food/dietarysupplements/ (accessed January 24, 2014).

8. Ibid.

of any contaminants are set extremely low—in some cases even lower than those permissible in pharmaceuticals. Often, an accredited third-party laboratory checks these products to verify the company's findings and attests to the purity of the product in a certificate of analysis (CoA). A reputable manufacturer will offer these documents to anyone upon request.

Prescribers of Chinese herbs are fully aware of the ways in which herbs act separately and together and how they may interact with Western medications. To avoid any adverse reactions, it is very important to tell your practitioner of Eastern medicine about all the drugs and other supplements you are taking. Providers are required to report any such reactions to the manufacturer and the Food and Drug Administration, along with the lot number and expiration date of the prescribed herb in order to isolate any contaminated batches or follow trends.

Patients also have a responsibility to use herbs wisely and treat them with the same respect as any pharmaceutical agent. Herbal formulas should be taken exactly as prescribed. More is not necessarily better. Prescriptions should not be shared with family or friends, any more than you would give someone else your Western medication. This is particularly true in Eastern medicine, where one disease can have many different causes. The cause of your disease may not be the same as the cause of your friend's disease, even if you have the exact same Western diagnosis. The correct treatment for your condition may be the wrong one for your friend and could result in serious side effects.

By combining common sense with best practices, manufacturers, practitioners, and patients can work together to ensure that Chinese herbs are used safely for the benefit of all.

With respect to acupuncture, the overall risks are small. It is possible to have some bruising or bleeding at the needle-insertion sites. Infection in these areas is possible but unlikely, in view of the use of sterile, single-use needles. Practitioners also swab the area with alcohol before the treatment. Because of the use of sterile single-use needles and mandated clean-needle technique, there have been no reported incidences of HIV transmission in the United States. The only documentation of a hepatitis B outbreak, noted in 1988, was traced back to a single practitioner who was reusing unsterile needles,[9] which is absolutely not standard practice in the twenty-first century.

Some practitioners of the past used permanent needles during acupuncture treatments. There were reports of needle migration with this sort of needle. In these cases, the needles shifted position and were found embedded into major organs or the spinal cord. This technique has been abandoned and is not currently used in the United States.

Rarely, a patient may experience the unpleasant sensation of "needle shock." In Western terms, this is a vasovagal reaction where the vagus nerve is stimulated and leads to a decrease in heart rate and blood pressure. The patient will feel clammy, nauseated, and faint. This reaction is easily treated by removing the needles, repositioning the patient, and needling or applying pressure to other acupuncture points. Needle shock is usually short-lived and not dangerous. It can easily be avoided through correct positioning and technique.

An even rarer complication is the puncturing of internal organs such as the lung or bowel. A properly trained practitioner takes measures to avoid this by using appropriate needling angle and depth. There are documented cases of patients with abnormal anatomy in whom these problems have occurred, but these are very unusual circumstances. In 2010, the US National Certification Commission for Acupuncture and Oriental Medicine reported that, in its forty-year history, there had been no deaths due to acupuncture among patients of licensed practitioners. Worldwide, it is estimated that there are fewer than two deaths per year due to acupuncture among tens of millions of patients. Serious adverse outcomes are almost solely associated with unlicensed or poorly trained practitioners.[10]

---

9. G. P. Kent et al., "A Large Outbreak of Acupuncture-Associated Hepatitis B," *American Journal of Epidemiology* 127 (3): 591–598.

10. National Certification Commission for Acupuncture and Oriental Medicine, "The Safety of Acupuncture and Oriental Medicine," www.nccaom.org (accessed January 24, 2014).

The National Institutes of Health consensus panel commented that the risk of complications from acupuncture is extremely low, frequently lower than that from conventional treatments. The same can be said of Oriental herbal medicine, according to the National Certification Commission for Acupuncture and Oriental Medicine.

Compare this with orthodox allopathic medicine. Other sources, such as the Institute of Medicine (now the National Academy of Medicine) and the Centers for Disease Control, estimate that conventional Western medicine is responsible for approximately two hundred thousand deaths per year, caused by complications from unnecessary surgeries, hospital-acquired infections, medical error, and non-error-related drug reactions. These deaths are classified as "iatrogenic," meaning they occurred in the course of medical treatment. In 2000, Dr. Barbara Starfield published a study in the *Journal of the American Medical Association* demonstrating that the annual rate of iatrogenic demise was the third leading cause of death in the United States, behind cardiovascular disease and cancer.[11] These are staggering statistics.

Why Should We Consider Integration of Eastern and Western Medicine?

Western medicine, for all its amazing technologies, has proven to be both expensive and, as we've just seen, risky. It does save lives in acute, emergency situations, but does little to improve the quality of life in chronic illness. Most of the ailments in our society are persistent in nature and caused by poor lifestyle choices. The strength of Eastern medicine lies in its ability to enhance the day-to-day functioning of the chronically ill through a combination of acupuncture, *tui na*, herbs, exercise, and diet. The integration of these two systems could improve medical care in the United States by decreasing complications and costs while increasing the overall health of the population.

---

11. Barbara Starfield, MD, "Is US Health Really the Best in the World?" *JAMA* 284 (4): 483–485, doi:10.1001/jama.284.4.483.

Americans are already using Eastern medicine in ever-increasing numbers. In 2002, the National Institutes of Health (NIH) conducted a survey of more than thirty-one thousand adults regarding their use of complementary and alternative medicines. By extrapolating the percentage of people who had used acupuncture as a healing modality, the NIH estimated that 2.1 million American adults had been treated with at least one component of Eastern medicine at that time.[12]

The survey was then repeated in 2007, and the results were very interesting. While the use of complementary and alternative medicines showed a very small increase in the intervening five years, the number of people who had used acupuncture had increased by 50 percent. It was estimated that 3.1 million adults and 150,000 children had been treated using acupuncture. Given the increasing demand that acupuncture services be covered by insurance companies, it seems that the trend is continuing.[13]

Eastern medicine has been shown to be safe, clinically effective, and fiscally cost-effective. It seems clear that adding these strengths to those of Western medicine can only result in better outcomes and healthier patients.

Are Western Physicians Willing to Incorporate Eastern Modalities?

In September 2011, the American Hospital Association released the results of a survey that stated that 42 percent of their member hospitals provided non-allopathic healing services, an increase from 37 percent in 2007. Approximately 40 percent of those services involved acupunc-

12. National Institutes of Health, "Complementary and Alternative Medicine Use among Adults: United States, 2002," http://nccam.nih.gov/news/camstats/NHIS.htm (accessed January 24, 2014).

13. National Institutes of Health, "Complementary and Alternative Medicine Use Among Adults and Children: United States, 2007," http://nccam.nih.gov/news/camstats/NHIS.htm (accessed January 24, 2014).

ture. Other available services that also fall in line with the Eastern philosophy of healing and health maintenance included lifestyle counseling, massage, and stress-relief modalities.[14]

On the educational front, over seventy universities across the United States are members of the Consortium of Academic Health Centers for Integrative Medicine. Among these members are such prestigious schools as Harvard, Tufts, Duke, Stanford, MD Anderson Cancer Center, the Albert Einstein School of Medicine, and the Mayo Clinic, to name but a few. These schools have acknowledged the importance of incorporating holism into medical care. Their students learn about the tenets and uses of Eastern medicine as well as other modalities such as Ayurvedic medicine, chiropractic, and massage. Although the students generally do not learn how to perform acupuncture or prescribe Chinese herbs, they gain an appreciation for the utility of Eastern medicine when combined with the standard biomedical care they have been studying.

These two fundamental changes in the education and practice of biomedicine demonstrate the willingness of Western physicians to collaborate with healers from other disciplines. Specifically with respect to Eastern medicine, there has been a stunning increase in its acceptance by allopathic health-care providers over the past two decades. In a survey performed in 1988, only 20 percent of Western physicians had a favorable opinion of Eastern medicine. When the survey was repeated in 2009, that number had exploded to 80 percent.[15] Given that statistic, it is safe to say that a great many Western physicians are genuinely interested in the incorporation of Eastern therapies into Western medical care.

---

14. American Hospital Association, "More Hospitals Offering Complementary and Alternative Medicine Services," https://www.aha.org/press-releases/2011-09-07 -more-hospitals-offering-complementary-and-alternative-medicine-services.

15. From the keynote address of the 2011 American Academy of Medical Acupuncture Symposium, given by Emmeline Edwards, MD, director of the Division of Extramural Research at the National Center for Complementary and Alternative Medicine, a component of the NIH, March 2011.

How Should I Approach My Doctor about Using Eastern Medicine?

Knowing that so many Western medical centers offer acupuncture and other Eastern practices such as tai chi and qigong classes, it is quite possible that your doctor may suggest Eastern medicine to you before you even have a chance to ask! But, if that doesn't happen, it doesn't necessarily mean that your physician isn't open to the addition of Eastern medicine into your treatment strategy. It could mean that your doctor doesn't know if Eastern medicine would be useful for your particular condition. Or they may not have access to reliable practitioners of Eastern medicine to whom they can send you. Or they may not want to suggest a therapy that might incur additional costs to you if your health insurance doesn't cover these services. These reasons should not prevent you from discussing treatment options with your doctor.

To have a meaningful discussion, you should come to the appointment prepared. You need to do a little homework. Since the inception of the internet, most physicians have been very comfortable with patients who have done some online research about their illness and are happy to go through the downloaded information with you. If you are going to present your doctor with such information, it is important that it has come from reputable websites. The World Health Organization report on acupuncture is a good place to start. You could also search the websites of several prominent medical centers that offer Eastern medical services and see what conditions they commonly treat.

You should call your health insurance company to see if Eastern medical services are a covered benefit and, if so, which providers are in the network. If this option is unavailable to you, you can cover the expense yourself, understanding that within three to five treatments you will know if they are beneficial. If you live near a school of Eastern medicine, there will be a community clinic where you can receive care for a reduced cost.

Now that you have determined for yourself whether Eastern medicine is a suitable modality for your condition and how you can access that care, you will feel more comfortable broaching the subject with your doctor. Generally, the situations in which patients explore options outside of biomedicine are those in which the patient is not improving. In cases where the problem is acute, Western treatment options usually solve things quickly. For patients with chronic conditions, healing may be slower and require greater effort on the part of the patient and the physician. Often both parties become frustrated with what appears to be a lack of progress. Eastern medicine is well suited to treat people in such circumstances. Some patients might worry that their doctor would be offended at the suggestion of a complementary therapy, but in truth, that rarely happens. Most Western practitioners are interested only in their patients' well-being and would be delighted at the prospect of successful treatment through Eastern medicine.

Occasionally, in difficult cases where a patient has not improved with conventional treatments, a physician may feel a sense of failure or embarrassment that they have not been able to help that person sufficiently. Following an honest and respectful discussion of Western and Eastern treatment options, often doctors and patients alike are relieved that a new plan has been formulated. Although the Western physician may not be administering the Eastern treatment themselves, they would still be a part of your health-care team and would certainly do their best to facilitate this new aspect of your care where possible.

It is very important that you keep your doctor aware of any non-allopathic treatments that you are undergoing. Even if you have decided on your own to seek the help of an Eastern medical practitioner, your Western doctor needs to know this, particularly if you are taking any herbs or supplements. Many medications can interact with herbs, supplements, and foods, leading to dangerous situations in which the action of the drug is either accentuated or diminished, possibly causing a medical complication.

How Should I Use These Two
Systems Together?

As in any good marriage, collaboration should be considered a dialogue between equals. In our experience, Eastern and Western practitioners who have the greatest success with the combined approach display respect for the abilities of their new partners and the strengths of the different medical systems. It is ultimately the patient who decides which intervention they will try, and in which order, but overall we feel that medical management should proceed along the following lines:

First, the patient should receive a thorough explanation of their condition, in both Western and Eastern terms. This may not occur during the same visit if two practitioners are involved. Whether in one appointment or two, the patient needs to understand what illness they have, its usual course, and its common complications.

Communication is key, not only between patient and providers but between the health-care practitioners themselves. It is important to find one of the growing numbers of Western physicians and Eastern practitioners who are willing to take the time to consult with each other. It is only through these discussions that the best solution for every patient can be found.

Next, each practitioner should carefully explain the treatment options, complete with a disclosure of risks. It is usually the risk profile of a treatment that will help the patient decide how to proceed. The patient can then weigh the risks and benefits of each option and determine the next best step. It only makes sense that someone would want to try acupuncture before back surgery, for example, because the risks of surgery are so much greater.

In many circumstances, Eastern and Western treatments can be used concurrently. In many musculoskeletal conditions, Western physical therapy can be overlapped with acupuncture treatments for a faster recovery overall. A patient can still stay on blood pressure medications, but can learn how to meditate to reduce stress and improve general well-being. A diabetic may be able to decrease their medication requirements by adhering to Eastern dietary therapy. Of course, any changes in medications should be strictly supervised by the conventional practitioner of the East/West pair.

It is very important to carry through with the treatment plan that is outlined by your Eastern and Western health-care providers. If you have pneumonia, you would complete the course of antibiotics that your Western doctor has prescribed. Similarly, you should follow the recommendations of your Eastern medical practitioner or you may not reap the full benefit of their expertise.

By now, you may be eager to start using this integrative approach to solve your health problems. The next step is acting on the knowledge you have gained by reading this book so far. It can be hard to change deeply ingrained habits all at once. Chapter 5 is designed to ease you through this transition. The upcoming topics, questionnaires, and "homework" provide the insights and skills necessary to create lasting health in the true sense of the word: physical, emotional, and spiritual.

Four Steps to Optimal Health

N OW WE ARE AT THE CRUX of the matter. In the preceding chapters, you have learned about the history of Eastern and Western medicine and how they can complement each other. You have seen how ancient concepts and practices lead to optimal health and how these transformations can be explained by modern science. You have a greater understanding of the powers at play within the American health-care system and what is at stake if the alarming epidemic of chronic disease continues to grow. You now have the tools to approach your primary care provider about incorporating the tenets of Eastern medicine into your care so that you reap the benefits of both healing systems. By blending the best of Eastern and Western medicine, you can attain true wellness—the maximization and balance of mental, physical, and emotional health.

But how do we put all that knowledge into practice?

To paraphrase an ancient Chinese proverb, "The longest journey begins with a single step." This applies to all of our endeavors. Some journeys are easier than others. If people are going to transform habits that are deeply ingrained, they must overcome a certain amount of inertia. We have been flooded with information about how to lead healthier lives, but putting all that excellent advice into action is the really tricky part. Not everyone can "just do it," as the popular advertising slogan instructs. If it were that simple, we'd all be in perfect health—focused, calm, slender, and fit. Most of us know what needs to be done, but do not take the necessary steps to achieve long-lasting results. The big question is, "Why not?"

In the last fifty years, Western psychologists have been studying how and why people make significant lifestyle changes. Initially, this may seem like just another Western reductionist way to pick apart a complex process, but the resulting theories and models have a great deal in common with Eastern medicine's approach to the patient. The predominant Western theory in this area is called the transtheoretical model of change, and it demonstrates what the Chinese have known all along: each person is a unique and multifaceted being who is traveling along on their journey at their own particular speed. Taking this into account, health-care practitioners are better able to tailor advice and interventions to meet their patients' needs.

The transtheoretical model of change was developed by Prochaska and DiClemente after they researched how people successfully made lifestyle changes.[1] They determined that when people make sudden behavioral changes without preparation, they commonly fail. Certainly some people can quit smoking cold turkey or exercise daily without missing a workout, but most of us need more preparation to make these significant shifts part of our routine. Prochaska and DiClemente discovered that long-lasting changes are more likely achieved if the person proceeds through five distinct stages:

Stage 1: Precontemplation (no intention of changing)
Stage 2: Contemplation (thinking about changing)
Stage 3: Preparation (getting ready to change within the next month)
Stage 4: Action (behavior change less than six months)
Stage 5: Maintenance (behavior change more than six months)

Variations include additional stages:

Stage 6: Relapse (regression to an earlier stage)
Stage 7: Termination (behavior has completely changed)

---

1. J. O. Prochaska and C. C. DiClemente, "Stages and Processes of Self-Change of Smoking: Toward an Integrative Model of Change," *Journal of Consulting and Clinical Psychology* 51 (1983): 390–395.

These last two stages may not apply to all situations. For example, some people never regress, and some behaviors cannot be completely terminated. While it is possible to quit smoking entirely, one cannot absolutely stop eating. Maintaining a healthy diet and avoiding overeating is a lifelong endeavor. In a similar vein, those who conquer addictive behaviors such as alcohol or drug abuse may always consider themselves to be in the maintenance stage.

Rather than achieving linear progression, most people progress through this model in a circular or spiral fashion. Very few people are able to modify undesirable behaviors on a permanent basis on their very first attempt. Often, they move between stages. This is perfectly natural and expected. The most important thing is to keep trying. Your persistence will eventually pay off, and you will find yourself transformed!

Another name for the transtheoretical model of change is the "stages of motivational readiness for change model." Use the questionnaire that follows to determine your current readiness for change; it will help you see from which stage you are starting. Then, based on your stage, you can use the exercises supplied in this book to assist you in moving from one stage to the next until you have achieved your goal.

When answering the questions in each survey or exercise, it is important to be completely honest. You might assume that just by reading this book you are past stage 1 (precontemplation) and are already in stage 2 (contemplation), but truthfully consider your circumstances. Did you pick up this book of your own volition? Are you eager to embark on your healing journey? Is a doctor or loved one nagging you to make lifestyle changes? Would you really rather stay as you are?

The word "change" in the questionnaire means any behavioral change you want to make. This could be anything at all, such as exercising, meditating, or being more attentive to your spouse. You can repeat this survey multiple times for multiple behaviors or over time to gauge your progress. For example, you may be an avid exerciser (maintenance stage) but you are still smoking and do not intend to stop (precontemplation stage). Keeping all of this in mind, start by completing the questionnaire.

Readiness-for-Change Questionnaire*

1. I intend to integrate this change into my life.   Yes   No

2. I have already integrated this change into my life.   Yes   No

3. I have been integrating this change for one to
   six months.   Yes   No

4. I have been integrating this change for more than
   six months.   Yes   No

SCORING

If you answered	You are in
1, No; 2, No; 3, No; 4, No	Stage 1: Precontemplation
1, Yes; 2, No; 3, No; 4, No	Stage 2: Contemplation
1, Yes; 2, Yes; 3, No; 4, No	Stage 3: Preparation
1, Yes; 2, Yes; 3, Yes; 4, No	Stage 4: Action
1, Yes; 2, Yes; 3, Yes; 4, Yes	Stage 5: Maintenance

*Adapted from B. H. Marcus, J. S. Rossi, et al., "The Stages and Processes of Exercise Adoption and Maintenance in a Worksite Sample," *Health Psychology* 11 (1992): 386–395.

Now that you have determined your readiness for change, you will be able to use the four steps for optimal health more effectively as you move toward your goal. Our four steps progress in a similar manner to the transtheoretical model:

- Step 1: Build a Positive Mind (Contemplation)
- Step 2: Set Your Goal and Plan (Preparation)
- Step 3: Start Your Action (Action)
- Step 4: Be Persistent (Maintenance)

Within the four steps are a series of exercises that will lead you from one action to the next. Tiny changes made over a long period of time are more likely to be permanent. These four steps can effectively help you reach your goal. Follow them consistently and you will definitely change your life!

Step One: Build a Positive Mind

It might surprise you to learn that before taking action to achieve improved health and well-being, we must first turn inward to observe the mind. A positive state of mind is paramount to your success, allowing you to carry through with any change you wish to make. It is the key to healing on all levels. Practitioners of widely varying systems of medicine, from Eastern to Western, have all noted the same thing: patients with a positive attitude generally heal faster and remain disease-free much longer than those who do not.

Our mind is a very special entity. It has tremendous power and can contribute both positively and negatively to our health. If used to create positive changes, the mind can help heal many illnesses, whether psychological, physical, or spiritual.

Changing the mind can change behavior; changing behavior can change health, relationships, and life circumstances. For example, a patient named Tiffani came to see me (Dr. Kuhn). She had extreme fatigue, muscle and joint pain, and many food allergies. She was unable to digest many foods, had insomnia, anxiety, depression, bowel problems, and was unable to keep weight on. She was 5 feet, 4 inches tall, but weighed only ninety-four pounds. Previously, Tiffani had seen at least ten medical professionals, including medical doctors, specialists, psychiatrists, psychologists, chiropractors, nutrition consultants, acupuncturists, and holistic MDs. During her search for medical help, she had changed her diet, taken medication and supplements, and been compliant with everything her doctors and therapists had prescribed, yet her condition did not improve. Her exhaustion and frustration brought her to my clinic.

I started treating Tiffani with acupuncture, herbs, and some supplements, but somehow Tiffani's improvements were not as great as I expected. Over time, and by listening carefully to Tiffani's concerns,

I realized Tiffani was not using her mind for healing at all. Her physical pain, along with her negative experiences and thoughts, were slowing her recovery. Tiffani's main frustrations were not being able to go out to eat with her family because she couldn't tolerate restaurant food, not being able to go shopping with friends because she would get sick in the store, and not being able to have friends over because she felt people didn't want to hear about her problems. Other frustrations included being unable to work or do things with her husband because she had no energy. All these limitations were creating relationship problems between Tiffani and her family and friends.

I encouraged Tiffani to take the first step and go out with her family. I explained that going out to eat is not just about food, but about keeping the family spirit going and keeping the family in harmony in a relaxed atmosphere. Even if all Tiffani could eat at the restaurant was soup, I was certain that Tiffani would have fun and enjoy being out with her loved ones. And she did! On the next visit, Tiffani told me what a great time she had had on that family outing. I prompted her to take the next step and call some friends to chat, keeping the conversation positive, and invite them out. These short excursions also yielded positive results.

I guided Tiffani, little by little, helping her remove her fears and frustrations in baby steps, cautioning her not to look for quick results. I explained that healing takes time, and if Tiffani felt too attached to the outcome of her actions, she might become more anxious and impatient. Tiffani overcame her reluctance and took positive steps almost every day. With each little thing she accomplished, she felt better and more hopeful. A few weeks passed, and her energy and attitude improved. Within another few weeks, her pain was reduced and she started eating more varieties of food, as her bowel problems had greatly diminished.

Encouraged and energized, Tiffani started going to my qigong classes. At first, she could not stay in class for more than fifteen minutes. After several weeks, she was able to stay for the whole hour. She then started to practice qigong at home, and soon she saw a tremendous improvement in her daily energy level and overall sense of well-being.

Later, Tiffani joined my tai chi class and absolutely loved it! Over the course of the following year, Tiffani maintained her new positive lifestyle and was able to start her own business.

Tiffani's story highlights how developing a positive outlook can be transformational. None of the amazing physical changes that Tiffani experienced would have occurred if she had not taken that first step. With guidance, Tiffani had an insight: she changed how she viewed eating out with her family. She was able to see what she could enjoy in that situation rather than what was lacking. The key to Tiffani's success was developing a positive mind.

A positive mind makes positive physical changes: relaxed muscles, reduced heart rate and blood pressure, balanced metabolism and blood sugar, and improved production of digestive enzymes. A negative mind produces negative physical results: tight muscles, irregular or fast heart rate, elevated blood pressure and blood sugar, low energy, poor metabolism, decreased enzyme production, and difficulty sleeping.

Some of these negative physical results had a purpose in the past. It would have been an advantage to have elevated heart rate, blood pressure, and blood sugar when running from a predator or combating a foe. This physical state, caused by the release of stress hormones such as adrenaline and cortisol, is known as the fight-or-flight response. It was instrumental to our survival as a species, but in modern-day life we do not allow ourselves to recover from these extreme episodes. We subject ourselves to many daily stressors, strive to meet sometimes unrealistic expectations, and often fail to nourish our bodies and minds. Physiologically, we are forever preparing for the next battle, just as our ancestors were; however, the constant secretion of these stress hormones can be detrimental to the body and the mind.

Your mind affects not only these physical elements, but also influences the social, behavioral, and interpersonal aspects of your life. It goes without saying that most people prefer the company of positive individuals. A positive mind involves love. Positive individuals often exude love. Love brings joy, healing, and happiness. Giving love and receiving love both arise from a positive state of mind. Love does not have conditions or bias. Love involves giving, selflessness, compassion, and kindness. Love produces healing results through a sense of inner peace. You love your family and your friends, but it is the love and compassion you give to yourself that will make the difference in your healing journey. It will allow you to develop a positive mind and lead a healthy life by quieting the fight-or-flight response and decreasing the release of stress hormones.

A positive mind that is calm and compassionate can help control emotions and cravings. This is why some people are better able to manage stress and achieve their objectives. A positive mind can improve your mental ability, concentration, and determination; however, other aspects are involved in reaching your goal.

Every action, such as altering habits, is predicated on making a decision to change and then actually carrying out that decision. A person's ability to follow through on resolutions can be influenced by many things. While many emotional components are involved, profound behavioral changes are not a matter of willpower alone.

From a Western perspective, making lifestyle changes requires not only desire and determination but also healthy brain chemistry. The compounds that convey messages throughout your brain and body are called neurotransmitters. Neurotransmitters are influenced by many factors, such as sleep patterns, exercise, nutrition, and meditative practices like qigong and tai chi.

Dopamine is the neurotransmitter that is released when you perform any action that results in a feeling of accomplishment. Any such pleasurable activity increases the secretion of dopamine. You can use this reaction to your advantage when trying to reinforce behavioral changes. Every time you complete a questionnaire or exercise in this book, reward yourself. The reward could be large or small. It may help if the reward reinforces the behavior you are trying to reinforce; for example, downloading great new music for your workout or purchasing a fancy kitchen gadget to prepare new, healthy recipes.

The purpose of the reward is to increase dopamine release. Then you will want to take the next step in your transformation. Pamper yourself with larger rewards for each accomplishment. If you never find time to read, curl up with a good book. If you love to paint, enroll in an art class. Play sports with friends, treat yourself to a movie, or purchase a new item of clothing. All these sorts of activities will release dopamine and you will want to continue on your healing path. Every time you reward yourself for performing a positive behavior, you will strengthen the association between that behavior and a feeling of well-being. You will reinforce positive, healthier habits.

Western neuroscientists have observed that positive reinforcement actually changes the way your brain functions. Using special magnetic resonance imaging studies called functional MRIs, it has been shown that people who practice this technique increase the number and activity of neural connections in various parts of the brain. They are, in fact, changing their mind. This property of the brain is called neuroplasticity, and studying it is altering the way conventional medicine looks at the brain, from both a physiological and psychological point of view.[2]

From an Eastern perspective, successfully making changes is a matter of common sense. Food, rest, activity, and self-reflection must be balanced to lead a healthy life. In today's hectic world, we may need some reminders about how to build a positive mind to achieve physical, emotional, and spiritual equilibrium. To this end, we have created a series of home study activities for building a positive mind.

The mind and body are intricately intertwined. Any variation in one aspect will cause changes in the other. This is why building a positive mind will have such an important impact on your body. The question is, what can you do to alter internal processes on such a deep level? There are three interconnected ways to approach this task:

- Change the way you *breathe*.
- Change the way you *think*.
- Change the way you *act*.

---

2. Norman Doidge, MD, *The Brain That Changes Itself* (New York: Viking/Penguin, 2007), 11.

The following pages are full of written exercises to guide you through this transformation. While some space is provided for short answers, we recommend you start a journal for daily entries. Your journal can be electronic or on paper. Remember to give yourself an appropriate reward for completing these homework assignments, which will reinforce your new behaviors, encourage persistence, and lead you to a state of true wellness.

Breathe

You may have noticed that some of the calmest, most centered individuals are those who engage in an activity that involves slow, deep breathing. These may be yoga practitioners, tai chi or qigong enthusiasts, or those who regularly meditate; maybe they only follow the habit of taking three deep breaths whenever they are upset. But the link between a tranquil demeanor and deep breathing is no coincidence: there is a direct connection between how breathing patterns are interpreted by the brain and the resulting emotion that a pattern will evoke.

Give this a try:

Start breathing very shallowly and rapidly for ten to twenty seconds. (Stop if you start to feel faint!) Notice how you feel, emotionally. Agitated? Anxious? Fearful? Describe your sensations here:

_____

_____

_____

Now take three long, deep breaths. How do you feel? Most people will say they feel calmer, more peaceful, or more relaxed. Write down your experience here:

_____

_____

_____

This association between breathing patterns and emotion has been demonstrated by a number of researchers, including Pierre Philippot. Philippot conducted an interesting pair of studies in which he showed that specific emotions evoke particular breathing patterns that usually occur when someone exhibits that sentiment. This pattern was consistent from person to person. He went on to show that the reverse is also true: when test subjects were asked to breathe in a particular pattern, they reliably stated that they experienced the associated characteristic emotion.[3]

Regulation of the breath is a part of many medical traditions and has been used for millennia to calm the mind and heal the body. From Tibetan meditation to the modern "relaxation response," from yoga to tai chi and qigong, the breathing techniques incorporated into these modalities can balance the sympathetic and parasympathetic nervous system through the modulation of neurotransmitters released in the body.[4]

Homework

Choose an activity that causes you to breathe in a pattern that allows you to feel both calm and alert. This could be qigong, tai chi, yoga, or meditation. It could be some other activity of your choosing. Pay attention to your emotions during these slow, deep breaths. It is OK if your attention wanders, as long as you keep coming back to your breath. Perform this activity for five to ten minutes each day, longer if desired.

Every day that you complete this homework, give yourself an appropriate reward. After several weeks, you will find that you won't need this reinforcement as often, if at all.

---

3. "Respiratory Feedback in the Generation of Emotion," http://www.scribd.com/doc/164856193/Respiratory-Feedback-in-the-Generation-of-Emotion-Philippot-2013 (accessed December 25, 2013).

4. T. M. Srinivasan, "Pranayama and Brain Correlates," *Ancient Science of Life* 11 (1-2): 1–6; D. Krishnakumar, M. R. Hamblin, and S. Lakshmanan, "Meditation and Yoga Can Modulate Brain Mechanisms That Affect Behavior and Anxiety," *Ancient*

Think

Thoughts and emotions are two different things. While they are inextricably linked, they are not the same. An emotion does not arise spontaneously. It is felt in response to a thought. It is not possible to change an evoked emotion, but it is possible to change the way you think.

So, how do you go about changing your thoughts? You challenge them. Take a step back and examine your thoughts about yourself and the world around you. Often our thoughts produce negative emotions such as fear and self-criticism. But is what you think really true? Are you exaggerating your situation, if only slightly? If your thoughts are true, then what? For example, say you are giving a big presentation at work. You know it is important. You might even get a promotion if you do well. You worry that if you botch it, your boss and coworkers will think less of you. You might even make yourself anxious thinking about it. But take a moment and challenge these thoughts. If your employee or coworker is giving a presentation and stumbles, do you think she is an awful person? Would you fire her? If you are working in an environment where this could be true, then consider how it is affecting your life and your physical and emotional health. It is certainly reasonable to acknowledge your nervousness before entering into a stressful situation such as public speaking, but with practice you can stop that emotion from generating a downward spiral of negative thoughts.

Use Your Fear

Fear is a double-edged sword. It can be a powerful motivator or a destructive force. Fear of blindness caused by diabetes can prompt you to control your blood sugars. Fear of a stroke might make you exercise and meditate to lower your blood pressure. However, fear that immobi-

---

Science of Life 2 (1): 13–19, doi:10.14259/as.v@i2il1.171; Michael M. Zanoni, "Healing Resonance Qi Gong and Hamanaleo Meditation," https://www.mikezanoni.com /meditation-qi-gong (accessed February 4, 2018).

lizes you is debilitating: it stops you from acting to prevent that which you fear. This in turn makes you more fearful. Being stuck in this vicious, unproductive cycle generates many negative physiological responses in the body and mind. You are forever in the fight-or-flight response, in a constant state of stress.

What would happen if you let this unproductive fear go? It is not easy to have a fear-free life, but it can be achieved through practicing mindfulness. Preparing answers and actions for things that could happen helps remove fear: preparing for the worst thing that could happen can help you be less fearful and less stressed. Through your actions, you may be able to avoid negative experiences, but if something really happens, you will know how to deal with the situation.

Homework

Ask yourself these questions and write down your answers:

1. What do I fear?

_____

_____

_____

_____

2. How likely is it that the things I fear will come true?

_____

_____

_____

_____

---

3. What steps can I take to prevent this from happening?

_____

_____

_____

_____

4. What steps will I take to improve my situation if these fears come true?

_____

_____

_____

_____

_____

Look for Solutions Instead of Complaining

It is human nature to complain. It is easy to get into a rut, complaining about a situation without making an effort to change it. Sometimes we have issues or problems from various life experiences. Instead of complaining, which can negatively affect ourselves and others, we need to try to find solutions.

Life is not always easy; that is part of learning. You learn to solve problems from adversity. Every time you find an answer or solve a problem, you feel a sense of achievement; you feel ready to take on the next challenge that lies ahead.

If you can look at a problem without fear, without attachment to the outcome, a solution will often present itself. The solution may not be complete—it may only be a step in the right direction—but it will alter the nature of your circumstances. You may think such a tiny shift is too insignificant to matter, but it is the accumulated momentum of individual small actions that creates the process of change.

Homework

Think of a personal problem that has been unresolved for a long time. Now think of the outcome you desire. Write down one or more ways that you could solve this predicament. At this point, there is no need to act on your ideas. Consider as many creative solutions as possible and write them down here:

_____

_____

_____

_____

_____

Find Something Positive in Everything

When you come across something negative, ask yourself, "What is positive in this situation?" Changing the way you think and looking for the positive aspects of a situation can improve your energy. When you look on the positive side of things, you allow yourself to heal. People who are always looking at the negative side of a situation can build a barrier to their healing path.

One of my (Dr. Kuhn's) patients cured her chronic headaches simply by changing her viewpoint from negative to positive. For many years, "Heather" had ongoing headaches that affected her life and made her fatigued all the time. When she started to see me, Heather mentioned that she had a lot of stress from both work and home. At work, she was a manager of forty people in a big corporation. She felt overwhelmed all the time and sometimes had to make difficult decisions. At home, her husband cared for their two young children, and Heather felt guilty because she was less involved in child care than she wanted to be.

Regarding her work-related stress, I asked, "Do you do the best you can at work?" Heather said yes. I explained to her that she should be satisfied with what she has done for the company because that is all she can do. Since she did the best she could, there was no need to feel stressed. Regarding Heather's home stress, I asked her, "Are your children and husband happy at home without you present?" She replied, "Yes, they are very happy." I explained to her that since they were happy, then she should be happy, not stressed. The breadwinner has to

---

Homework

It is not easy to be positive all the time, but it can be achieved by daily mindful practice. Whenever you have a negative experience, write down one positive aspect of that encounter below. For example, you are given a task at work that involves learning new procedures. It may take more time and effort at the beginning, but eventually you have mastered a new skill that you can add to your résumé.

_____

_____

_____

_____

_____

_____

---

work to provide the others with comfort and necessities. Heather was making herself ill by thinking of things in a negative way. Soon after she understood this and saw the positive side of her situation, Heather's headaches were greatly relieved and were almost all gone within several days. As Heather continued to view her situation in a positive light, her headaches resolved, her energy improved, and she became happy both at work and at home.

Be Thankful

Many cultures around the world devote certain holidays or special occasions to giving thanks for whatever comforts they have in life. Some years these comforts may be few, but there is always something for which to be grateful. Appreciation and gratefulness are a part of many religions. A sense of thankfulness to some higher power, something outside ourselves, can change our outlook for the better.

It really does not matter if you are religious. It is not about organized religion; it is about spirituality. Having a belief system that incorporates regular expressions of gratitude has many healing benefits. Various researchers have documented the positive effects of articulating appreciation.

Emmons and McCullough demonstrated that a study group that, on a daily basis, wrote in a journal about things, people, or situations for which they were grateful noted superior life improvements than those in groups assigned to chronicle their problems or how they were better off than others. The life improvements noted in members of the grateful group included increased "alertness, enthusiasm, determination, attentiveness, and energy." They also reported being able to exercise longer, sleep more deeply, and stay asleep for greater periods of time.[5]

---

5. R. A. Emmons and M. E. McCullough, "Counting Blessings versus Burdens: Experimental Studies of Gratitude and Subjective Well-Being in Daily Life," *Journal of Personality and Social Psychology* 84 (2003): 377–389.

The above benefits were not simply the subjective impressions of the study participants. When friends, family members, and colleagues were asked to describe grateful individuals, such individuals were more likely to be rated as happier, helpful, optimistic, and trustworthy.[6]

Expressing appreciation and gratitude decreases the release of stress hormones and increases hormones such as serotonin, which balance your nervous system. You will feel calmer, more optimistic, and more motivated. With this kind of reinforcement, you can move forward with ease.

Homework

Every day for the next month, write down one thing that you appreciate or for which you are thankful. You will likely need to use your journal, but just to get you started, write down three experiences for which you are grateful:

_____

_____

_____

Always Have Tomorrow

We all feel down or unwell from time to time. Tell yourself, "Tomorrow I will feel better." It is true; the next day is different. We all have ups and downs, rainy days and sunny days. We sometimes feel overwhelmed, frustrated, and have bad experiences. If we keep thinking about these negative feelings, we can feel stuck with these pessimistic moments.

---

6. M. E. McCullough, R. A. Emmons, and J. Tsang, "The Grateful Disposition: A Conceptual and Empirical Topography," *Journal of Personality and Social Psychology* 82 (2002): 112–127.

Our energy can be depleted. If we tell ourselves, "Tomorrow will be a better day" or "Things will change tomorrow," we don't feel as frustrated, and we feel calmer instead.

Our brain gets rest overnight. Often our troubles seem smaller in the morning. Daily meditation also calms the brain and allows you to approach a problem refreshed and clear-headed. Being able to take a step back, whether for a ten-minute pause to meditate or a full night's sleep, allows you to see things in a more positive light.

Act

Now that you are changing the way you breathe and think, it is time to act. There are three actions you can take to build your positive mind:

1. Forgive

2. Reach out

3. Change your dynamics

Forgive

The first and most important action is to forgive. The first and most important person to forgive is yourself. We all have regrets and imperfections, but everyone can improve and make changes. If you can forgive yourself, you can forgive others. This is a type of mindfulness practice that can be incorporated into, and assisted by, regular meditation.

If you don't forgive, you are holding on to negative energy, and the negative energy can make you sick. Forgiving can assist healing and is also part of healing. Forgiveness can be toward anyone or everyone. Forgiving is not the same as excusing, condoning, or forgetting wrongful behavior. It is possible to forgive someone for morally "unforgivable" acts. If you choose to forgive someone who has harmed you, that person's underlying behavior or character may not change. By choosing to forgive, you are changing the relationship dynamics and taking steps to end the control that person has over your well-being. Practicing forgiveness can eliminate resentment and be a powerful motivation for people to move forward, be happy, and heal.

Homework

1. If you feel you have been wronged or have hurt another person, think about whether the situation has affected your physical, mental, or spiritual health. Describe these symptoms here:

   _____

   _____

   _____

   _____

2. Choose to forgive or ask forgiveness from the person or people involved. If it is not possible to speak directly with these individuals, write a journal entry or note (which you may or may not decide to send). In one or two sentences, without accusation or excuse, give or ask for forgiveness here:

   _____

   _____

   _____

   _____

3. Understand that this process may take time. As you forgive others or receive forgiveness, notice how your physical, mental, or spiritual state has changed. List these transformations here:

   _____

   _____

   _____

   _____

(continued)

4. If you are having difficulty letting go of resentment or grudges, you may want to seek the help of an unbiased friend or relative, spiritual counselor, or medical professional. List at least three trusted individuals here and arrange a meeting as soon as possible.

_____

_____

_____

_____

Various studies over the last decade have shown that the act of forgiving can have positive health benefits, both physical and emotional. These include lower blood pressure, lower risk of alcoholism or substance abuse, less anxiety, and better relationships with others.[7]

By being compassionate, forgiving yourself and others, you can bring balance to the part of your nervous system that controls the fight-or-flight response. Self-compassion has even been associated with decreased inflammation and protects against inflammatory and autoimmune diseases.[8]

While doing these forgiveness exercises,[9] you would do well to remember the famous words of St. Augustine: "Resentment is like taking poison and hoping the other person dies."

7. Mayo Clinic, "Forgiveness: Letting Go of Grudges and Bitterness," http://www.mayoclinic.com/health/forgiveness/MH00131 (accessed December 25, 2013).

8. J. G. Breines et al., "Self-Compassion as a Predictor of Interleukin-6 Response to Acute Psychosocial Stress," *Brain, Behavior, and Immunity* 37:109–114. pii:S0889-1591(13)00537-0, doi:10.1016/j.bbi.2013.11.006.

9. Mayo Clinic, "Forgiveness: Letting Go of Grudges and Bitterness," https://www.mayoclinic.org/healthy-lifestyle/adult-health/in-depth/forgiveness/art-20047692?pg=2 (accessed January 6, 2018).

Reach Out

Many people are afraid to reach out, but developing social connections and a sense of community can have many benefits. By reaching out, you learn from others: you get positive energy and support. You also have the opportunity to contribute to your social network, which will increase your own feelings of belonging and self-worth.

By seeking out social relationships, you may even increase your life expectancy. Researchers at Brigham Young University performed a meta-analysis of 148 studies, involving over three hundred thousand people. This study showed that over a seven-year period, social relationships decreased the risk of dying by 50 percent. It did not make a difference whether you had a preexisting medical condition, whether you were male or female, or even whether you were young or old; stronger social relationships predicted a longer life.[10]

To put it another way, the risk of low social interaction is equivalent to other well-known health risks such as smoking fifteen cigarettes a day or being an alcoholic. Being socially isolated is more harmful than not exercising and twice as harmful as being obese.

Homework

1. At least once a week, contact an old friend or talk to a colleague about something other than work. List these contacts here:

_____

_____

_____

_____

(continued)

---

10. Julianne Holt-Lunstad, Timothy B. Smith, and J. Bradley Layton, "Social Relationships and Mortality Risk: A Meta-Analytic Review," July 27, 2010, http://www.plosmedicine.org/article/info:doi/10.1371/journal.pmed.1000316#s4.

2. Every week, schedule a social engagement with a close friend or casual acquaintance. It could be as long as a day at the beach or as short as a quick coffee after work. List these outings here:

_____

_____

_____

_____

3. Join an organization of people with whom you share a common interest. For example, if you play a musical instrument, join a community orchestra. If you enjoy sports, join a local league. If you like ethnic food, take a cooking class. Write down six group activities and do the one you would enjoy the best.

_____

_____

_____

_____

4. Volunteer your time at a community institution of your choice, like the Humane Society, a food bank, or your public library. Write down six organizations in your area and offer your help to the one that interests you most.

_____

_____

_____

_____

Reaching out to others will not only help you build a positive mind, but will also help extend your life!

Change Your Dynamics

You can change your dynamics both internally and externally. So far, the homework you have done is helping you change your internal dynamics and build your positive mind. An important attribute of a positive mind is an open mind. When you keep an open mind, you are more likely to try new experiences and meet new people. Every new encounter will stimulate your brain and make changing your old routines much easier.

Let's look at a common situation: many people do not like their jobs. They feel like they have to do their job just to pay the bills. That is not healthy; saying "I hate my job" will decrease your energy. If, instead of saying "I hate my job," you say, "I learn from this job no matter what," your energy changes. This will change the energy of the working environment, and you may find amazing results.

For example, say hi to every single person you meet at work. If you are usually disorganized, then make a plan for each workday. If you micromanage your colleagues, call a brainstorming meeting about an issue that needs to be solved, and let your colleagues run with their ideas. Buy a cup of coffee for a person you usually hesitate to talk to; invite a coworker to lunch, or take a walk together. You may not hate your job anymore because you are more open-minded, willing to try new approaches, and have changed the energy in your work situation.

Now push yourself to change your dynamics outside of work. Take a different route home. Sample new foods. Pick a radio station at random and listen to it for a while. All these shifts in your routine cause your brain to stop running on autopilot and pay attention to your inner and outer environment. When you are truly aware of what is going on around you, your brain creates new neural pathways. By changing how you act, you can change the way you think; you are more likely to feel inspired, energized, and ready to meet life's challenges.

Even though you have reached the end of step one, remember we are never fully finished building our positive mind. You may want to revisit some or all of these pages during your journey toward true wellness as a reminder to breathe, think, and act with compassion, optimism, and gratitude.

Step Two: Set Your Goal and Make a Plan

A goal without a plan is just a wish.

—Antoine de Saint-Exupéry

Goal-setting is beneficial in many endeavors: succeeding at school, running a business, leading a company, teaching, financial planning, and achieving optimal health. You know what you want to achieve, what is important to you, what you need to improve, and what kind of life you want to have. When you know yourself, setting a goal is easy, but to achieve a goal requires effort and planning.

Setting a right goal is better than setting a big goal, but any goal is good as long as you can achieve it. Let's begin with a small goal. Once you achieve it, you can set another goal. Achieve one goal after the other, and after you achieve whatever goal you set, you know you can achieve anything.

In healing, every little step or improvement you want to make can be a goal. If you have a cholesterol problem, you can set a goal to get your blood cholesterol to normal in one year, or even three months. Then you will do whatever you can to regulate the cholesterol level. You will change your diet, increase your exercise, and eliminate alcohol. If you want to lose weight before summer comes, you will eat healthy and light: avoid going out to eat too frequently, do daily exercise, and remove junk food and sweets. If you want to feel less pain from your fibromyalgia or arthritis, do therapeutic exercise daily, eat the right foods, or take some herbs to assist in healing.

Nothing can happen without effort. You may need to change your daily routine, change eating habits, and change lifestyle. All these require mindful practice and determination, but once the new routine is established, it becomes easier and almost effortless.

Whatever goal you want to reach, you will need to make a plan. A plan can help you organize your behavior pattern. Making a health plan or healing plan can be different for each individual because each one of us has a different reason for healing: losing weight, healing a chronic physical issue, healing an emotional issue, or having a better relationship with someone, for example. Everything has a cost, even a behavior that is in your best interest. Starting an exercise regime will take time away from other activities. Giving up cigarettes may make you feel uncomfortable socializing with friends who continue to smoke. Eating more fruits and vegetables may increase your grocery bill. Only you can decide where the tipping point lies. That is the point at which you will progress from thought to action.

Complete the following chart by identifying a behavior you wish to modify. List all the pros and cons that come to mind. If there are more cons than pros, you must address the cons in order to move forward. The homework exercises at the end of this section will help you in this regard.

	Pros	Cons
Behavior		

Now that you know what you want to accomplish, you can determine how to succeed. You need to design a healing plan.

Let's say you want to exercise more, and your goal is to run a marathon. Most people cannot do this without a plan. You need to create a training schedule, acquire the correct equipment, and improve your diet to meet your increased nutritional needs. Making so many changes all at once is quite daunting. A lot of people would find it so overwhelming that they would simply give up.

Sudden large changes are often unsustainable. This is why many individuals fail to alter habits that are damaging to their health. The best way to avoid this pitfall is to make these changes little by little. Think of yourself as an infant learning to walk with baby steps, one foot at a time. If you really do want to run a marathon, you must honestly assess your current exercise tolerance and gradually increase your time, distance, and intensity. Your first baby step might be only a walk around the block, but that's OK! Remember: your health should be your priority. You want these changes to last a lifetime.

In her superb book *The Four-Day Win*, Martha Beck likens these small changes to the adjustments that are made while navigating a sailboat. The sail settings are fine-tuned to alter the course of the boat. It may seem as though a tiny variation will not make a difference, but over time and distance, the effect is huge! She advocates making one small, rewarded adjustment after another to create lasting change. Although her book is primarily about weight loss, she dovetails the transtheoretical model of change with the Daoist philosophy of moderation and compassion to prepare readers to achieve their goals.[11]

In the homework for this section, we invite you to continue your journal, completing the following exercises. You are in the preparation stage, refining your unique plan to attain health and well-being. The key to moving through this step and arriving at the action stage is being able to identify and remove barriers to your success. Keep this in mind while you are completing these exercises.

Homework

In your journal, answer these questions. You can answer them all in one session or break it down to one question per day. Continue to give yourself appropriate rewards for completing the homework and accomplishing any steps you need to take in preparation for moving to the action stage.

1. What is your primary health concern? You may have several problems you wish to solve, but start with the one that is most important to you.

(continued)

---

11. Martha Beck, PhD, *The Four-Day Win: End Your Diet War and Achieve Thinner Peace* (New York: Rodale, 2007), 145.

2. What is your goal? Try to be specific. For example, "I want to control my diabetes by consistently keeping my blood sugars within the recommended range over the next month."

3. What is the solution? Continuing with the diabetes example: "I will eat less refined sugar, exercise more, and take my medications (if prescribed)."

4. What are the steps you need to follow to reach the above solution? This is one of the most important parts of creating your plan.

You need to gather a lot of information to develop a realistic plan that will yield results. If you want to get your diabetes under control by decreasing your intake of refined sugars, exercising more, and taking your medications, you need to make an honest assessment of your current knowledge and habits. What foods do you eat now? Which contain refined sugars, and what foods would be better substitutes? Can you think of ways to resist the temptation to eat foods that will excessively elevate your sugars? How do you politely decline well-meaning people who insist you try their dessert? What sort of exercise do you like? What intensity of exercise are you currently capable of performing without injuring yourself? When and where are you going to exercise and with whom? Regarding your medications, do you forget to take them? Are they easily accessible? Do they have side effects that discourage their use?

Breaking down each step like this may seem daunting, but it will give you a lot of insight into how you make changes in your life and why you may not have succeeded in the past.

Write down the steps you are going to follow, making sure that the steps are practical; otherwise, they will be more difficult to accomplish. Do not be ashamed to write down what you may consider to be a ridiculously small change in your habits. As Martha Beck points out, it is the stacking of a series of tiny adjustments that will take you where you want to be. The title of her book *The Four-Day Win* refers to the number of days she recommends implementing a change before making another alteration. For each day, you should give yourself a small reward and a slightly larger reward on the fourth day. In her book, she describes how she became an avid exerciser. Her first four-day win consisted of driving to the gym and sitting in the parking lot for three minutes for four consecutive days. Yes, she did reward herself. For the next four days, she went into the gym and pedaled on a stationary bike for three minutes. Over a period of about three weeks, she came to enjoy and benefit from longer and more vigorous exercise sessions.

This is exactly how you should be approaching your goal. Baby steps, consistently applied, will get you much further than an all-out sprint that you cannot sustain.

5. What are the obstacles you have faced in the past?

Many people have failed because they had some obstacles they did not recognize or they were not able to overcome. Obstacles can be work or living situations, time constraints, even friends and relatives.

In keeping with our diabetes example, a recognized obstacle might be this: "Aunt Sally brings me a dozen home-baked cinnamon rolls every Sunday. I eat them all because I don't want to appear rude or hurt her feelings. After that, it takes me the whole rest of the week to normalize my blood sugars."

Once you know the obstacles, you will be practicing mindfully to rise above them.

6. How will you overcome these obstacles?

Sometimes this is the most difficult part, especially if your obstacles are people you love. You have to be creative and find solutions. Perhaps you can eat a small piece of Aunt Sally's cinnamon rolls and share the rest with friends. Maybe Aunt Sally doesn't understand the seriousness of your condition. If you asked for her help, she would most likely give it. Suggest that you and

(continued)

she spend time together baking, but use less-refined, healthier ingredients.

Whatever the obstacle, there is usually a solution. No time to exercise because you have kids? Take them walking with you, ask a friend or relative to babysit on a regular basis, or trade off childcare with another parent.

Consider substituting an enjoyable activity for an unhealthy one. For example, if you are handy, use that skill to supplant a bad habit. Knit, paint, or make jewelry instead of lighting up a cigarette. Take up woodworking, learn an instrument, go Latin dancing—anything you have always wanted to try.

7. How will you organize and document your healing plan?

These days, there are innumerable electronic and paper organizing systems. You may think these are a waste of time, but people who write down their goals and document their efforts have a greater chance of reaching their target. Choose which system works best for you, but be diligent and use it daily.

It doesn't have to be a fancy device either. For example, most people have a calendar hanging on the wall. All you need to do is to put healing hours on the calendar for each day. Regardless of what kind of work you do or how busy you are, you can make anything happen if you have written information on the calendar and read it daily. You can put down your diet menu, daily exercise hours, or any other important things you have to do.

Many of these systems use a worksheet format, which allows you to write down all the small steps you need to take to reach your goal, giving you a roadmap to follow. You can include your daily physical goals, and you can set mental or emotional goals.

Once you have done all your homework, set your goals, identified obstacles to implementation, and created contingency plans, you might find a checklist useful. Relying on a checklist makes life easier. You have already done your prep and made all the hard decisions. Now, follow your checklist as faithfully as possible. Many high-tech, high-stakes industries, including hospitals and airlines, use checklists. Checklists improve safety and efficiency. Checklists get results. Checklists also capitalize on the sense of satisfaction we get from crossing off something on our to-do list. Biochemically, this is a little rush of dopamine that rewards your brain for performing a desired behavior. This is how you develop healthful habits, and a checklist can help. To that end, we have supplied you with a template for your True Wellness Checklist that you can modify to suit your dietary preferences. See appendix C.

By combining your journal with the True Wellness Checklist, you will have a unique how-to manual for your journey to optimal well-being.

Step Three: Start Your Action

Now that you understand why and how, it is time to start your action and make things happen. We all have different plans even though we have similar goals. We must put theory into action. Without action, nothing works. As unique as each of us is, as individually tailored as each healing plan might be, there is one item that should be on everyone's list: exercise.

Moving your body should be included in your daily routine. Our body is made of many parts, similar to a machine that is made of many components. Think of a machine that is not used regularly: it can rust, its parts becoming stiff and unmovable. Our body is similar. It needs to move to prevent stiffness and poor function.

It doesn't matter what kind of exercise you do; as long as you exercise, it gives you benefits. You should choose whatever exercise you like so that you will do it consistently. People have many choices of exercise: jogging, walking, going to the gym, playing sports, dancing, aerobics, yoga, tai chi, qigong, and martial arts. But in fact, no matter how good people say a particular exercise is, you won't do it if you don't like it. You need to find the right ones for you.

Generally speaking, most Western exercise promotes blood circulation, whereas most Eastern exercise promotes energy circulation. Both are very important in preserving good health and preventing illness. One type of exercise might be better than another type for some people, but not for everyone. We are all different, so we choose different exercises.

Eastern Exercise versus Western Exercise

Eastern-style exercise works on an internal level, whereas many Western exercises work on an external level. "Internal level" means intrinsic energy that may not be measurable. "External level" means aspects that are measurable: for example, elevated heart rate, increased respiration, more muscle mass, and firmer muscle tone. Here we are using the term "Western exercise" to describe cardiovascular exercise. Eastern martial arts certainly improve cardiovascular fitness. No matter the type and style, you should choose whatever exercise you like and do it regularly.

Here are some differences between Western exercise and Eastern exercise:

Western Exercise

- A Western workout improves muscle mass and muscle tone but does little for flexibility.
- Western exercise can improve circulation by increasing both heart rate and breathing rate.
- Movements are typically fast, heavy, and vigorous.
- Western exercise focuses more on external energy.
- Western exercise places more focus on the physical body and less on the mind.
- Age may be a limiting factor; people may have fewer choices as they get older.
- There are some restrictions for people who have certain medical conditions.

- Western exercise can be used for health maintenance, stress management, and prevention, therefore increasing longevity.
- Younger people are more likely to participate.
- Western exercise is more yang; it is more dynamic and forceful.

Eastern Exercise

- Eastern exercise improves energy circulation, flexibility, and muscle tone.
- Eastern exercise improves circulation by improving fundamental internal energy.
- Movements are slow and gentle, suitable for all ages and abilities; you are benefiting and feeling good emotionally, mentally, and physically.
- Eastern exercise requires proper breathing and mental focus.
- You can practice anywhere; no need for special equipment or special clothing.
- Eastern exercise improves posture and balance.
- Eastern exercise is fun to learn and sometimes challenging, which is great for preventing brain aging.
- As you get older, instead of losing your abilities, they may improve; tai chi and qigong are perfect examples of this.
- With practice, Eastern exercise benefits mind and body; it is a great exercise for stress reduction.
- Eastern exercise includes preventive work, improving organ function, assisting in healing, and promoting longevity.
- Eastern exercise is more yin; it is more calming and restorative.

People often ask, "How do these exercises fit in our lives? With so many beneficial exercises, how do I find time to do them all?" People do yoga, aerobics, weightlifting, and other forms of exercise. But after hearing so many good things about qigong and tai chi, especially for healing, they have a problem finding time to do it all. We recommend that you pick your priority for the day, but over the course of each week maintain a balance between Western and Eastern exercises to obtain maximum cardiovascular, musculoskeletal, and neurological benefits.

Benefits from Qigong and Tai Chi

A practice session can be as short as five or ten minutes a day, or it can be longer. Qigong and tai chi practice benefits all parts of the body, including all the organ systems and the brain.[12] In the following section, we discuss some examples of these benefits.

Cardiovascular Benefits

Qi is dynamic. It performs like a motor that pushes the blood where it should go. If a person's qi is strong and circulates well in the body, their blood will also circulate well. If a person's qi is stagnant or weak, it will cause blood stagnation, which according to Eastern medical theory can cause heart disease. Qigong and tai chi contribute to better heart health by regulating the autonomic nervous system. In particular, these exercises activate the vagus nerve—which is a great way to preserve heart energy, normalize cardiac arrhythmias, and maintain normal blood pressure.

Respiratory Benefits

Through deep and slow breathing, more oxygen goes into the lungs. Slow and deep breathing also activates the parasympathetic (calming) part of the autonomic nervous system. Recall that the nervous system interfaces with the immune system. This process helps the functioning of all cells through proper oxygenation as well as improves defensive energy—which in Western medicine we call the "respiratory immune system"—through modulation of the immune system. The lining of the nose, throat, lungs, gut and urinary tract all contain immunoglobulin A (IgA). IgA is an antibody in the respiratory tract, which protects it

---

12. Dr. Aihan Kuhn, *True Brain Fitness: Preventing Brain Aging through Body Movement* (Wolfeboro, NH: YMAA Publication Center, 2017), 11.

from various germs and pathogens and acts as the first line of defense against bacteria and viruses. If the respiratory immune system is strong, immunoglobulin A (IgA) can fight germs, allowing less chance for colds and other respiratory infections to take hold. This is why those who practice tai chi or qigong generally have fewer illnesses.

Gastrointestinal (GI) Benefits

Both tai chi and qigong can improve stomach and spleen energy, which is related to digestion and absorption. From a Western perspective, tai chi and qigong regulate the vagus nerve, which also controls digestion. With regular practice, digestive enzymes and digestive movement stay balanced through vagus nerve regulation.

Musculoskeletal Benefits

Once the circulation of the qi and blood are improved, muscles receive more oxygen and blood—the muscles become more resilient, more toned, and stronger. Muscle aging is delayed, and joints become more flexible. Overall, we can maintain a younger body even though we are going through the aging process.

Weightlifting develops muscle strength and muscle mass more than qigong or tai chi do, with the exception of exercises related to martial arts with weapons. Qigong practitioners rely on qi (energy) rather than their muscles, and qi is just as effective as muscle strength.

Nervous System Benefits

Qigong offers huge benefits to our nervous systems, both central nervous system and peripheral nervous system. Qigong helps concentration, improve mental alertness, helps to control emotion, and keep body is ordinary shape. Practice also helps to preserve vision and hearing as the body ages.

Metabolism and Endocrine System Benefits

Balanced qi also helps balance the body's organ systems, which helps balance metabolism and the endocrine system. Qigong practitioners rarely have hormonal imbalance and poor metabolism. Here again, these benefits are due to the effect that qigong and tai chi have on our nervous systems. The central and peripheral nervous systems are intimately connected to the endocrine and immune systems. Neuroendocrine-immune dysfunction can explain a variety of Western diagnoses such as chronic fatigue syndrome, also known as myalgic encephalomyelitis.

Immune System Benefits

Qigong and tai chi maintain normal immune function.[13] We have already spoken about how these exercises can improve respiratory immunity to keep infections at bay. For cancer patients, a healthy immune system can prevent infections during treatment. For those without cancer, a healthy immune system can identify precancerous cells and destroy them.

By balancing the sympathetic and parasympathetic nervous systems, qigong and tai chi also balance the immune system, so that the immune system is neither too weak nor too strong. A weak immune system will result in recurrent infections. An overly aggressive immune system may result in autoimmune diseases like rheumatoid arthritis. In autoimmune diseases, the immune system turns against the body and attacks normal tissue. Qigong and tai chi help keep the immune system balanced.

Other benefits of Eastern exercise include delayed aging, improved balance, reduced risk of falling and injury, and improved memory.[14]

Engaging in both Western and Eastern exercise is important for maintaining our healthy lives. Neither is superior to the other: they complement each other, balance each other, and are equally valuable.

---

13. Dr. Aihan Kuhn, *Simple Chinese Medicine: A Beginner's Guide to Natural Healing and Well-Being* (Wolfeboro, NH: YMAA Publication Center, 2009), 137.

14. For further reading, please see "Recommended Reading and Resources" at the end of this book.

Qigong for Daily Nourishment
Quick Warm Up

1. Turn Body

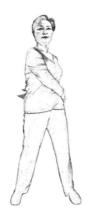 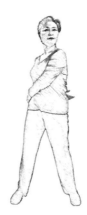

Feet are shoulder width apart.

Swing your body from left to right, right to left. Allow your arms to follow your body, swinging side to side. Repeat 16 to 32 times.

2. Shake Hands

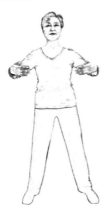 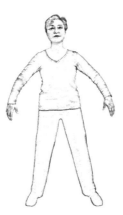

Keep the same body posture. Shake both hands upward and downward in front of your body.

Relax your arms and body while you are shaking your hands.

3. Shooting Star

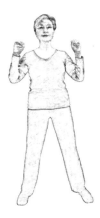

Bend your elbows so that your hands raise up to the sides of your shoulders. Keep your elbows pointed downward and your hands in a light fist. Quickly throw your hands upward and open your fingers. Repeat 16 times.

4. Reach Sky, Touch Earth

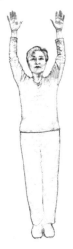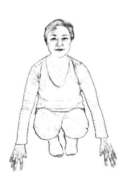

With your feet together, raise your hands up with fingers pointed upward.

Bend your knees and touch your hands to the floor. Roll your body back up to a standing position. Repeat this 8 to 16 times.

5. Knock the Body

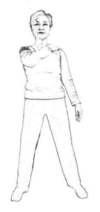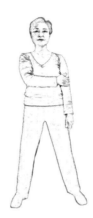

Gently knock your body with an open palm: use the right palm to knock the left upper chest, left arm, left shoulder. Repeat 3 times, then change sides.

Use the left palm to knock the right upper chest, right arm, right shoulder. Repeat 3 times.

Take a deep breath.

Daily Short Qigong Practice for Busy People

1. Open to See the Sky (Open All Channels)

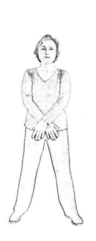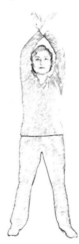

Raise your arms in front of your body and above your head as you inhale; separate your arms, then lower them down along the side of your body as you exhale.

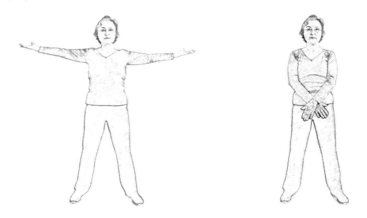

Again, raise your arms in front of your body and above your head as you inhale; lower your arms down along the side of your body as you exhale.

If you have neck problems, you may modify this exercise as follows:

When your arms are raised, turn your head toward your left hand. As you lower your arms, allow your head to move as your eyes follow the movement of your hand. The second time you raise your arms, shift your gaze to your right hand. As you lower your arms, allow your head to move as your eyes follow your right hand.

Repeat this movement 4 times on each side.

2. Reach Feet

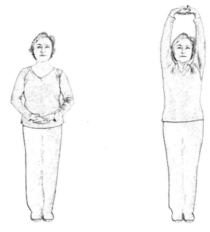

Interlock your fingers and raise your arms up above your head as you inhale.

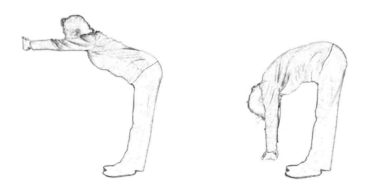

Bending forward with your arms still extended, touch the floor; relax the upper body and arms while taking three deep breaths.

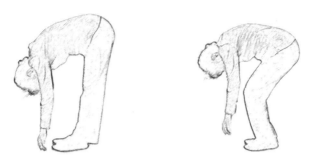

Slowly roll your body up, returning to a standing position. Repeat this movement 4 times.

3. Moving Qi through the Body

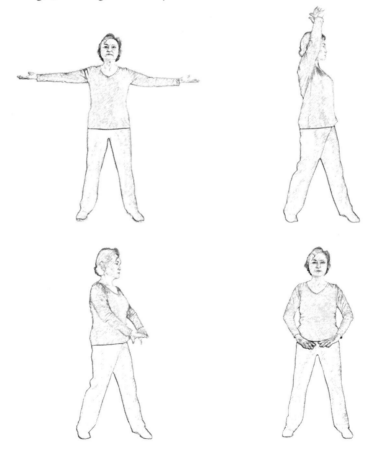

Take a deep breath as you raise your arms up along the side of your body, then above your head; at the same time, turn your body to the left, keeping your arms extended. As you exhale, slowly turn your body to the center, at the same time slowly lowering your arms down in front of your body, palms down. (It will look as though you are pressing something down in front of your body.) Inhale as you raise your arms up along the side of your body, then above your head; at the same time, turn your body to the right, keeping your arms extended. As you exhale, slowly turn your body to the center, at the same time slowly lowering your arms down in front of your body, palms down.

Inhale and raise your hands up along your back. When your hands reach chest level, move your arms to the front of your body. Exhale and press your hands down, at the same time bending forward until your fingers (hands) touch the floor. If you cannot reach the floor, you can place your hands on your ankles or shins. Hold this position for three breaths, then slowly roll up while taking a full breath.

The above two movements make one set.

Repeat this for a total of 4 sets.

4. Connect Heaven and Earth

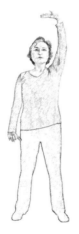
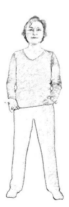

Feet are shoulder width apart. Starting with your hands in front of you, at the level of your lower abdomen, turn your left hand palm up and keep your right hand palm down. Inhale and raise your left hand up as high as you can, at the same time pushing your right hand downward as low as you can; exhale and relax both hands, moving your left hand down and letting both hands meet in front of your lower abdomen.

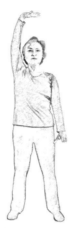

Now turn your right palm up and your left palm down. Inhale and raise your right hand up as high as you can, at the same time pushing your left hand downward as low as you can. Exhale and relax both hands, moving your right hand down and letting both hands meet in front of your lower abdomen.

Repeat these movements 8 to 16 times (4 to 8 times on each side).

5. Bring Qi to Three Dan Tian

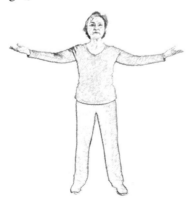 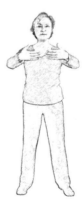

Inhale as you move your arms out to your sides at shoulder level. At the end of the inhalation, hold your breath for a count of three. Exhale as you move your hands to the upper Dan Tian, which is your upper chest (heart and lung area). At the end of the exhalation, hold your breath for a count of three. Repeat this movement 3 times.

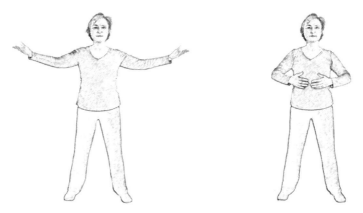

Inhale as you move your arms out to your sides at shoulder level. At the end of the inhalation, hold your breath for a count of three. Exhale as you move your hands to the middle Dan Tian, which is your stomach area. At the end of the exhalation, hold your breath for a count of three. Repeat this movement 3 times.

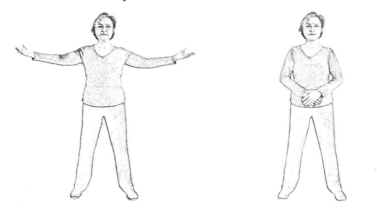

Inhale as you move your arms out to your sides at shoulder level. At the end of the inhalation, hold your breath for a count of three.

Exhale as you move your hands to the lower Dan Tian, which is your lower abdomen (reproductive organs, large intestine, small intestine). At the end of the exhalation, hold your breath for a count of three. Repeat this movement 3 times.

6. Qi to Five Senses

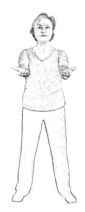 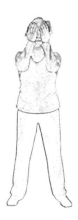

Raise your hands in front of your body and inhale. Slowly exhale and move your hands to your eyes (without touching your eyes), and hold this position for three breaths. Inhale and move your hands away from your eyes.

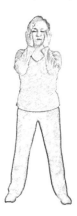 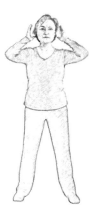

Exhale as you move your hands over your face (without touching your face), and hold this position for three breaths. Inhale and move your hands away from your face; exhale and move your hands over yours ears (without touching them). Hold this position for three breaths. Relax your arms and body with another breath.

Repeat this series of movements 3 times.

7. Dancing Saturn

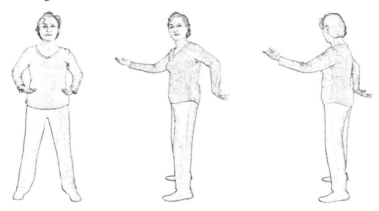

Put your hands at your waist with palms facing up. Turn your body to the left while circling your left arm back, circling the right arm from right to left in front of you at the same time the left arm is circling back. Then turn your body to the right while circling your right arm back, circling the left arm from left to right at the same time the right arm is circling back. Repeat, turning the body to the left, circling the right arm from right to left, at the same time the left arm is circling back. This exercise is a constant motion with both arms alternately circling inward at waist level. Do this 16 times (8 on each side).

8. Push Boat

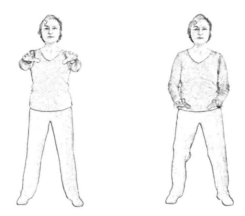

Inhale as you raise your arms to shoulder height in front of your body. Exhale as you gently press your arms down.

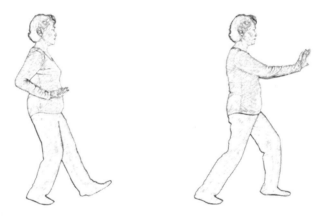

Step forward with your left foot, with heel down, at the same time moving your hands to chest level, palms facing up, and inhale. Exhale, turn your palms to face forward, shifting your weight onto your left foot, with the whole left foot on the floor. At the same time, push palms forward in the same direction as your shifting weight. Inhale as you shift your weight back onto your right leg and bring your hands back to waist level; exhale as you repeat the forward foot motion, pushing your hands forward. This will feel as though you are rocking forward and back. Repeat this sequence 8 times.

After 8 repetitions, change legs, step forward with your right leg, and repeat the same movement sequence, shifting your weight forward onto your right foot and backward onto your left foot.

Ending

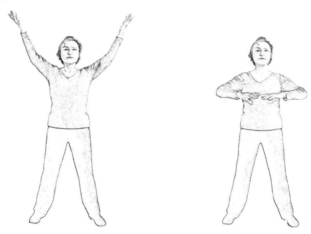

Start with the Y pose. To perform the Y pose, inhale and raise your arms up and apart to form a Y.

Hold the Y pose for three breaths. On the third exhalation, gently lower your arms in front of your body.

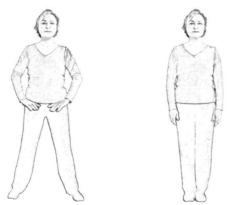

Focus your mind to connect energy from heaven to earth. Receive energy from heaven into your fingertips, through your hands, arms, body, legs, and feet, connecting energy to the earth.

General Principles for Eating Well
Diet in the USA

The diet in the United States is very out of balance for the majority of the population. People eat too much meat, too many sweets, too much dairy, and too-large quantities of food. Junk food is very common in many households. Row upon row of processed foods line our supermarket aisles.

It is all right to eat fast food once in a while, but too many people rely on fast food for at least one of their daily meals. If our job involves a lot of physical work, that diet might be okay, because physical work can burn off those extra calories. But in America, a majority of occupations involve sitting to do computer work or performing other deskbound jobs. In this case, we have to change our diet. In addition, since most people do not make time to do exercise, the accumulated calories, along with the chemicals in the processed food, can cause weight problems. Poor nutrition and eating habits have been linked to many illnesses such as heart disease, high blood pressure, cholesterol problems, diabetes, liver disease, bowel diseases, digestive disorders, and cancer. Here are some general principles of a balanced diet:

- Eat foods with a variety of colors.
- Eat foods with a variety of flavors.
- Eat foods that are properly balanced for your energy.
- Add spices to your food.
- Eat smaller quantities and include a variety of healthy snacks.
- Eat less meat and more vegetables and fruits; beans and rice are a good source of protein.
- Instead of a typical North American diet, eat more ethnic foods, especially Mediterranean cuisine.
- Reduce sweets and junk food.

Quality and Quantity

A proper diet also includes the right quantity of food and the right quality of food. The right quantity will not make your stomach too full;

half full is the signal that you should think it is about time to stop eating. The right quality means you should try to eat more homemade, healthy, and delicious meals.

How we eat also affects our health. One common issue is that many workers, such as teachers, nurses, and shift workers, have only thirty minutes for a lunch break. They have enough time to shovel food into their mouths, and don't even taste it. This kind of eating habit is not good for the brain or for the body. Eating too quickly does not allow the brain to sense when the stomach is full. The biochemical signaling that occurs between the stomach and the brain is not in sync, allowing people to overeat. Then digestion becomes difficult and can cause abdominal pain and distension.

Supplements

People often ask what supplements they should take. This is a tough question, because every patient is different, with a different underlying constitution. Generally speaking, if you are active, exercise regularly, eat well, eat a variety of foods, are in good physical shape, and have a good energy level, a good mental and spiritual state, and sleep well, you may not need to take supplements. You are probably getting enough nutrients for your body to function properly.

You may benefit from supplements if you have an underlying medical condition or if your diet is extreme and causes imbalance of nutrition and energy. What kinds of supplements a person should take depends on what kinds of problems they have. For example, if you don't eat enough fruits and vegetables, you need to take a multivitamin with minerals daily. If you don't eat enough multigrain breads or cereals, you need vitamin B complex, especially B1. From an Eastern perspective, if you have an organ energy imbalance or blockage, supplements may not work because they will not be thoroughly digested and used by the body. For mild energy blockages and imbalance, simply adding appropriate exercises will help supplements work much better. For major blockages and imbalances, you may need to get treatment such as acupuncture, *tui na* therapy, or Chinese herbs prescribed from a practitioner.

For particular disease entities, Western research has shown that certain supplements are very beneficial. You should speak to your health-care provider about nutritional support for your condition or request a referral to a nutritionist.

Water

Many people don't drink enough water. Water is very important in maintaining bodily functions and metabolism. Many people ignore water intake, some because they are too busy, others because they are unaware of its importance. When they feel sick or not well, they don't relate these feelings to lack of water.

Water makes up most of our body, especially our brain, which is more than 80 percent water. If a body becomes dehydrated, a person may have various symptoms such as headache, dizziness, poor metabolism, fatigue, and feelings of stress or anxiety; they may experience reduced muscle tone or muscle cramps, and become prone to kidney stones. Water helps the kidneys flush out toxins in the body, so being continually dehydrated allows these toxins to accumulate. People often ask me (Dr. Kuhn), "How much water is enough?" During regular weather, the body should get eight glasses of water daily. In the summer, the body needs eight to ten glasses of water a day depending on whether the person is outdoors (where he or she sweats more) or indoors with air conditioning. Another consideration is whether a person's job is physical or sedentary. Overall, let thirst be your guide. You will become thirsty with as little as a 1 percent drop in your body's total water stores, but this is not dangerous. It is a warning signal that you need to drink.

Coffee

Drinking coffee in moderation does no harm to the human body, but if people drink too much coffee, it can cause health problems. Coffee can affect digestion and cause stomach problems if it is overconsumed. Because of coffee's effect on the absorption of calcium and other minerals, it can also play a role in osteoporosis. Coffee may also cause pain for people with fibrocystic breasts or an inflamed urinary bladder. One to two cups of coffee is enough. If you are regularly drinking more, you should consider changing this habit. Choose to drink more water or other healthy beverages instead of coffee.

In step 3, Start Your Action, we made recommendations about the actions you should take on your path to optimal health. To help you keep track of your actions, you may use the True Wellness Checklist in appendix C. This checklist is a summary of important actions that research has shown will improve your health:

- moderate cardiovascular exercise and resistance training
- regular qigong practice
- regular meditation practice
- adequate consumption of fruits, vegetables, nuts, legumes, and water
- adequate sleep

Step Four: Be Persistent

It does not matter how slowly you go, as long as you do not stop.

—Confucius

From ancient philosophers to modern psychologists, every thinker in every age has described what it takes to be successful. They often agree that it helps to be talented, intelligent, or even just plain lucky. But when they get right down to it, the main ingredient of any successful endeavor is persistence. Persistence is the ability to work at a task consistently in spite of boredom or setbacks. It is the capacity to try and try and try again in the face of adversity. This effort will lead to steady change over time.

Persistence is one of the keys to successful healing. Often, people can initiate life changes, but have difficulty maintaining them. Every New Year, resolutions are made—plans to improve our health, strengthen our relationships, increase our productivity in our chosen profession. Usually, during the first couple of weeks, we are enthusiastic and keep to our plan, then gradually we may become less consistent in our efforts.

Sometimes the forces that disrupt our new routines are external. We get sick, so we can't exercise. We have a work deadline, so we don't find the time to meditate. Our family needs more of our attention, so we stop journaling. At other times, the problem is internal. We procrastinate, we rationalize, or we just can't seem to summon up the discipline it takes to complete the task at hand.

This is where the "just do it" mentality comes in. Developing persistence does require daily discipline to act on the plan that you have created. Discipline feeds persistence and persistence reinforces discipline. Every day that you perform a component of your action plan, you are gaining momentum and developing persistence. It is important that you do something every day that moves you closer to your stated goal, and it is even more crucial that you do not get derailed if you temporarily lose focus. Once in a while everybody chooses to skip the gym. Or chooses cupcakes over broccoli. Or chooses late-night TV over sleep.

The key word here is choice. We all make choices. We are faced with dozens of choices every day. It is the sum total of each individual choice that determines whether you progress toward your goal. The key to developing persistence is choosing to do what is necessary to achieve that goal each time you are at a crossroad. Do you hit the snooze button, or do you get up and meditate? Do you surf the internet for an extra fifteen minutes, or do you practice qigong? Over time, the majority of your choices must advance your cause or you won't realize your objective. That is not to say that you won't want to lie in bed for a few minutes more sometimes, and that's OK—it's your choice. You may have a few days, or weeks, or even months, when you feel that you are back at square one. You may feel that you have relapsed and are accomplishing less than you had hoped. This is a normal part of the process of change.

Remember that in the transtheoretical model of change, relapses are expected. People tend to move through major life changes in a spiral fashion, shifting from the maintenance stage to the relapse stage, then back to the contemplation or action stage. Eventually, you will stabilize in the maintenance stage if you consistently make choices that further your goal.

Still need more motivation? Try the exercises below.

Homework

1. Think about the reasons you chose to start down this healing path. Consider how this issue has contributed to your suffering. Who, besides yourself, is affected by the problem you are trying to solve? What could happen if you stop following your action plan? What could happen if you reach your goal? Write your answers here:

_____

_____

_____

_____

2. Set up a buddy system. Do you have any friends, relatives, or coworkers who might want to join you on your journey? Many people find it easier to share their goals and action plans with other people. Going to a tai chi class or trying new recipes together not only helps you achieve your objective, it also builds strong social connections that are vital to optimal health. Think of three people who may share your health concerns and invite them to participate in a suitable activity. Document the results here:

_____

_____

_____

_____

_____

3. Practice qigong and/or meditate daily. Qigong and meditation improve your clarity of mind and can increase your resolve. For one week, describe how you feel after these practices here:

(continued)

_____

_____

_____

4. Avoid distractions. Our modern world provides many distractions, particularly electronic ones. These devices can be real
   time-wasters. They divert your attention away from activities
   that will enhance your health and eat away at your ability to
   persistently pursue your goals. Identify the distractions in your
   life and write down the times you choose a distraction over a
   more healthful activity. Decide what needs changing and how
   to implement those changes.

_____

_____

_____

_____

5. Create habits. We are all creatures of habit; we can use this fact
   to our advantage. Once you choose to establish a healthy
   routine, you are more likely to continue it, because you don't
   have to make that same decision every day. If you are having
   trouble maintaining all the healthful habits you would like,
   choose one and spend time working it into your daily schedule.
   Write your chosen habit here and be sure to incorporate it into
   the True Wellness Checklist (see appendix C).

_____

_____

_____

_____

Many people can start something but are not able to keep up with it. For instance, every year in January, the gym in every city is full, since many people sign up to keep a New Year's resolution. This resolution could be to get fit or lose weight. As the months pass, the number of people at the gym starts to drop, leaving a trail of broken resolutions.

One of the keys to successful healing—or to the success of anything—is to be persistent. To be persistent, discipline is needed. People who have discipline can usually get from A to Z. Discipline feeds persistence and persistence reinforces discipline.

We live in a modern world, facing new things every day: new techniques, new machines, new software, new programs, new stores, new websites, new technologies, new drugs, new everything. We are distracted often, and we often forget fundamental stuff: keep things simple and keep focused. Persistence requires focus, and focus helps us make better decisions, making life less chaotic and a lot easier.

For people with chronic issues, the first question to ask yourself is, "How did I get this?" The next question is, "How can I get better?" When you ask these questions, you are on your way to finding answers. This is a positive practice. As we discussed previously, looking for answers to these questions will help you find solutions, set goals, and make a plan. You can start your actions, whatever they are. Then, the tricky part is, "How can I be persistent?"

In healing, the incentive to be persistent is, "I don't want to suffer anymore. I don't want to feel this way anymore." The ones who can take charge of their own health will most likely improve their health, and the ones who rely on doctors or other medical professionals may have lingering symptoms. I (Dr. Kuhn) have seen many people develop discipline after a health crisis such as a heart attack, stroke, or cancer diagnosis. They know they may not survive if they don't change their lifestyle, diet, and activities, and then continue to persistently live that way.

Persistence needs to have the right attitude and a positive mind. Persistence needs a special way of thinking: "I am a special person, so I can do this." That is true. It takes a special person to do things persistently. Once you develop a routine, your persistence becomes easier. A routine of self-healing can help you become a healthy, happy person and can save your life. By making physical and mental exercises a regular habit, you can dramatically improve your health, decrease your medications, and feel good instantaneously. More important, these daily exercises improve your clarity of mind and strengthen your resolve to stay on your healing path.

We are all creatures of habit. We can use this fact to our advantage. Once a healthy habit is well established, we are more likely to continue the routine.

Making small changes over time will ultimately bring optimal health. This concept applies to all components of a healthy lifestyle. Again, from a Western perspective, research has shown that small behavioral changes that are rewarded will cause the brain to create new neural pathways and establish new habits. This demonstrates that the brain can change. You do not need to feel stuck in old habits. The newer Western theory of brain plasticity will give you the hope that change is achievable, and persistence is the key.

Conclusion

Dao, Healing, Success

EASTERN CULTURE EMPHASIZES MODERATION, balance, equilibrium, and being one with nature. Our planet Earth and our bodies are part of the same cosmos: if our planet were to lose balance, there would be consequences. There is no doubt that our climate has changed, and all of us have experienced recent chaotic weather patterns. In medicine, disease trends have changed too—from infectious diseases to degenerative diseases. With the discovery of antibiotics, fewer people die from infection. Instead, death is more likely from the diseases caused by a modern lifestyle, such as heart disease, stroke, diabetes, liver disease, and cancer. This is the result of our changing lifestyle: from more physical work to sedentary work, from whole foods to processed foods, from the consumption of minimal sugar to excessive sugar, from adequate sleep to chronic insomnia. From the Eastern perspective, sitting too much, indulging in dietary indiscretions, and getting inadequate sleep can cause qi and blood deficiencies and stagnation, and these can lead to all kinds of illnesses. From a Western perspective, sitting too much, indulging in dietary indiscretions, and getting inadequate sleep can lead to obesity, diabetes, hypertension, heart disease, joint pain, and even cancer. Either way you look at it, our modern lives lack balance.

Any system that is out of balance will start to malfunction sooner or later. This applies whether the system is mechanical or biological. Many people take good care of their cars. They use the correct formulation of gasoline, they stop and start smoothly so as not to wear out the parts, they take their car in for regular servicing. All this is to ensure that the car is using fuel efficiently and functioning optimally. Some people take better care of their cars than they do of themselves.

When your energetic systems are out of balance, you will also start to malfunction. To avoid this disequilibrium, you must supply your body with nutritious food, obtain adequate amounts of restorative sleep, conduct your life at a pace you can sustain, and commit to regular self-care. Self-care includes calming your mind, moving your body, seeking professional help when needed, and strengthening connections to your family, friends, and community.

Eastern medicine is a special medical healing system that uses multiple natural methods to bring a body into balance and achieve optimal health. Eastern medicine can be used to treat specific diseases, but it is really designed to be used before you get sick. To paraphrase another ancient Chinese saying, "Taking medicine when you are ill is like digging a well after you are thirsty." Eastern medicine strives to prevent disease.

For those people already suffering from an illness, Eastern medicine can provide tremendous relief. It is very complementary to Western medicine. We have seen people get much better results when using both forms of medicine in the treatment of many complicated conditions, including cardiovascular disease, diabetes, and cancer.

This book has been devoted to seeking a balance between two great medical traditions, showing the similarities and differences, the complexity and simplicity of each. The goal of both Western and Eastern medicine is to help you live fully, to manage your energy wisely. A life of optimal health may not be entirely free of illness, but our intention is to show you ways that you can blend the best of these healing systems to minimize suffering and maximize your well-being.

In chapter 5, step 1, we encouraged you to work through various exercises to develop your positive mind. These exercises involved examining and perhaps changing the way you breathe, think, and act. These three steps do not need to be restricted to cultivating your positive mind. By taking the time to breathe, think, and then act, you can enrich every aspect of your life. We feel strongly that this process will positively reinforce every change you wish to create on this journey. With that in mind, we would like to reiterate these principles:

Breathe

There is no question that breath control plays a large part in our health. The physical and emotional benefits have been documented in many research papers that involve conditions as varied as asthma, multiple sclerosis, stroke, anxiety, and depression, to name but a few. Various medical systems incorporate breath control for energy management, pain relief, improved sleep, and mental alertness. Breathing exercises that are tied to meditative practices have been used for millennia. Qigong and tai chi both focus on the breath. I (Dr. Kuhn) have spent decades guiding people to optimal health by teaching them qigong and tai chi. I am so committed to qigong, tai chi, and the way of the Dao, that I will continue to teach these techniques and principles to my patients and students until my last breath.

Tai chi and qigong, along with yoga, are used for preparation for meditation, which has been shown to have numerous positive effects, including reducing stress, decreasing blood pressure, and subsequently decreasing the risk for heart attack or stroke.

Whether for three minutes or thirty, or somewhere in between, meditative breathing is strongly encouraged as a daily practice.

Think

The universe has two forces: the yin force and the yang force. These two opposite forces constantly balance, support, and control each other. A sunny day follows a storm. Winter follows fall, and spring follows winter. If anything is extreme, consequences result; the old passes away and the new comes. A bad day is always followed by a good day. These facts cannot be denied, ignored, or twisted. This is the way of the world. Everything has two sides: the positive and the negative. Nothing is perfect. You need to look at the positive side of things and not let the negative parts bother you. If there are too many negatives in your life, then you know you need to make some changes internally.

To build a balanced life, you need to think about the positive and practice letting go of the negative. Focus on the present. Only if you are able to let go of the past are you able to focus on the present. This is easier said than done. You need to constantly tell yourself to let go of the things that bother you and whatever is not natural for you. Daoist practice is different from Western practice. Western psychotherapy encourages you to talk about your feelings, fears, and past, or whatever is in your mind. It is helpful to give people the chance to let things come out, but it does not help them to let go. Every time you talk about the things that bother you from the past, you replay these negative images in your mind, and reinforce the negative memory. Daoism teaches you to not hold on to these negative things. Let go of what no longer serves you. Focus on the present and your hopes for the future, so you can move on to a new day, a new and better-balanced life.

In ancient Chinese culture, Daoist practices have a big impact on a person's life, including in healing. I (Dr. Kuhn) noticed that Daoist practice is starting to be recognized, and more people use it for self-improvement. I have personally benefited greatly from learning and practicing the Dao, and I organize a monthly study group to help others heal.

Daoism teaches us to think differently—to go with natural forces, not against them. Daoism teaches us to be simple: more spiritual, less materialistic. Daoism teaches us to relax our mind and our body, to balance our energy and our life. The more we relax, the more we can learn and heal. People who understand and practice Daoism seem to have much happier and healthier lives.

Daoist practice definitely helped me let go of things that have no value for my health. For work, it helps me relax, see things clearly, and find direction easier. There were times when I used to be confused when making decisions, but not anymore. I know my direction, and I know how to get there. With Daoist practice, and tai chi, I am able to connect with my inner spirit and allow my inner spirit to guide me to enjoy my life and to contribute to my community. But best of all, it has made me a very strong person.

You too can let go of past fears and troubles by following the principles of Daoism. By creating balance in your life, you can focus on the task at hand—assessing your current health situation and planning your healing routine. Think of ways to use your energy efficiently by identifying and minimizing obstacles, creating checklists and schedules, and doing extra research if you wish. We invite you to make use of the Resources and Recommended Reading section for more in-depth study of the topics we have discussed.

Act

When Dr. Martin Luther King Jr. addressed an assembly of students, he encouraged them to create a blueprint for their lives, to have aspirations, and to set goals. But he cautioned them that all this thinking and planning meant nothing if it was not followed by action. He urged them to start the process by doing whatever they could, no matter how seemingly small the step, saying, "If you can't fly, then run. If you can't run, then walk. If you can't walk, then crawl. But whatever you do, you have to keep moving forward."

We recognize that everyone moves forward at their own pace, and may even go backward or sideways! The important thing is to make a shift in a better direction. Each small positive change creates a ripple effect and gathers enough momentum to make the next small positive change possible. This is how the upward cycle begins—one step at a time.

This is the point at which you choose your path. Only you can act on the information that you have gathered about your own health and well-being. How will you now utilize your energy? How do you want to live your life? Have a frank discussion with your health-care provider about any problems you may have and ask for their recommendations. Consider adding other modalities to your care—acupuncture, massage therapy, personal training, health or life coaching, psychotherapy. Assemble your own health-care team. Whatever it takes to keep you on track to optimal health!

As you move forward you will see that more than your individual health hangs in the balance. You will be a role model for those around you. Your friends, your parents, your coworkers, and your children will all notice the positive changes that you will achieve in your physical, mental, and emotional health. You may inspire others to tackle their own health concerns. More important, you may encourage others, particularly the children in your life, to adopt habits that will prevent them from falling ill in the first place. This is the only way to solve this country's health-care crisis. The current system cannot cope with the ever-increasing chronically ill patients with diabetes, heart disease, obesity, digestive problems, and mental health concerns, to name but a few.

You can make a difference. You can be an equal partner in your care. When I (Dr. Kurosu) was near the end of my gynecology residency, I spent a considerable amount of time training with one of the senior attending physicians, Dr. John Morgan. I noticed that when giving instructions to his patients at the end of each visit, Dr. Morgan would emphasize the components of care that they, themselves, could control. He would say, "You can solve your own problem." This was not meant to be dismissive. He was clear that he would help them in any way he could, but that certain aspects of the solution required the patient's commitment to healthier behaviors. Dr. Morgan displayed every confidence that the patient would be able to achieve those goals. His patients left the office feeling empowered, knowing that Dr. Morgan trusted them to act in their own best interest.

We both feel strongly that the patient and the health-care provider must work as a team. Think of the times that you have had successful interactions with a medical professional. There may have been some commonalities. Were your unique insights into your condition acknowledged? Were you given enough time to have your questions answered? Were you involved in the decision-making process? Were you offered the support and tools necessary to be actively involved in your care, to "solve your own problem," as Dr. Morgan would say?

Wherever possible, there must be a balance between what the practitioner does for you and what you do for yourself. Your input matters. Engagement in your own healing creates equilibrium within this partnership. We hope that by reading this book and completing the exercises, you have new insights into your health concerns and have been able to create stronger relationships with your health-care providers, both Western and Eastern.

No matter where you start your journey, if you pay attention to your breath through meditation, qigong, and tai chi; carefully examine your thoughts; and create a healing plan, the actions you take will change your life. These actions will include feeding your body well, exercising regularly, managing your stress, and improving your relationships. These practices and behaviors affect the neurology, gene expression, and biochemistry of the body. All the exact mechanisms and pathways may not yet be known, but thousands of researchers around the world are gradually discovering why these modalities are effective in restoring health and preventing disease.

In your quest for true wellness, keep an open mind and take advantage of all that Western and Eastern medicine can offer. You will blaze your own trail to optimal health.

Breathe. Think. Act.

Developing Through Discipline

In embracing the one with body and soul,
Can you be undivided?
In controlling your vital breath,
Can you be supple as a newborn child?
In cleansing your inner vision,
Can you make it flawless?
Can you love and lead the people,
Without cunning?

In opening and closing the gateway to heaven,
Can you be like the female?
In seeing all things clearly,
Can you be without erudition?
Bearing and nourishing,
Bearing without possessing,
Rearing without ruling,
This is the mystic virtue.

—from the *Dao De Jing* (spelled *Tao Te Ching* in many translations)

Acknowledgments

D R. KUHN AND I DEEPLY APPRECIATE the efforts of everyone at YMAA Publication Center and Westchester Publishing Services. At YMAA, we are indebted to publisher David Ripianzi and managing editor T. G. LaFredo, for their trust, guidance, and astute insights that enhanced the flow and format of this book. Many thanks also go to Tim Comrie who, as book production manager, diligently kept this project moving forward; Axie Breen, for her inspired cover design and drawings; and Barbara Langley, for her work as publicist and for educating us about the intricacies of that art.

At Westchester Publishing Services, we would like to acknowledge editor Deborah Grahame-Smith for shepherding us through the production schedule, and copyeditor Susan Campbell for her meticulous corrections and excellent suggestions that greatly improved the manuscript.

To Drs. Holly Olson and George Rozelle, we would like to extend our sincere thanks for writing forewords to this book. We do appreciate the demands on your time and are honored that you both considered this endeavor worthwhile.

Personally, I would like to thank Dr. Aihan Kuhn for her invitation to co-author the *True Wellness* series. Her encouragement and advice through the writing process has been invaluable. I am enormously grateful for the opportunity Dr. Kuhn has given me to advance the integration of Eastern and Western medicine.

I am grateful to Dr. Olson for her trust in allowing me to integrate acupuncture to her patients' care. To my own patients, past and present, I would like to express my appreciation for your confidence in my best efforts, which I hope were more a help than a hindrance.

No practitioner of any form of medicine emerges from training completely adept at their craft. Over the years, I have been most fortunate to learn from some incredible teachers, starting in medical school, then through internship and a residency in obstetrics and gynecology at the University of Toronto. More recently, I appreciate the education I received at the Institute for Clinical Acupuncture and Oriental Medicine in Honolulu. I am grateful to all my colleagues, of all disciplines, who were willing to share lessons learned over years of practice. In particular, I would like to thank Darcy Yent, ND, LAc, for starting me on this integrative path; Dr. Joseph Helms, for creating the certification program for medical acupuncture and furthering its cause; and Michael M. Zanoni, PhD, LAc, my teacher and practice partner, for being so generous with his wisdom and expertise.

Last, but far from least, I would like to send sincere gratitude and love to my husband, Rob, and daughter, Hannah, for sharing me with this ongoing project. I realize it has taken countless hours from our time as a family, and I thank you for that gift.

An Anti-Inflammatory Diet

Anti-inflammatory Pyramid

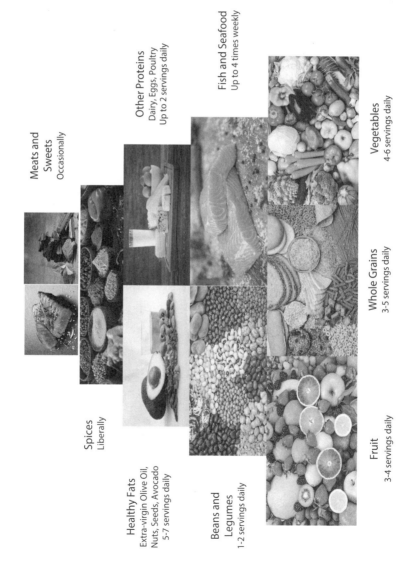

Meats and Sweets
Occasionally

Other Proteins
Dairy, Eggs, Poultry
Up to 2 servings daily

Fish and Seafood
Up to 4 times weekly

Vegetables
4-6 servings daily

Spices
Liberally

Whole Grains
3-5 servings daily

Healthy Fats
Extra-virgin Olive Oil,
Nuts, Seeds, Avocado
5-7 servings daily

Beans and
Legumes
1-2 servings daily

Fruit
3-4 servings daily

Illustration courtesy of Shutterstock

Glycemic Index and Load

THE GLYCEMIC INDEX is a measure of how quickly a food is digested into simple sugars within a specific time. The index uses a standardized amount of white bread as its reference point because white bread is metabolized very quickly and causes sudden increases in blood sugar levels. One slice of white bread is assigned a value of 100. The glycemic index compares how an equivalent amount of other foods affect blood sugar levels in the same amount of time. The glycemic index of a food is assigned a number between 1 and 100, based on how quickly it raises blood sugar values compared with white bread. For example, an apple has a low glycemic index value because it causes a lower rise in blood sugar levels compared with white bread in the same amount of time. In general, low, medium, and high glycemic index (GI) values are grouped as shown here:

Low GI < 55
Medium GI = 56–69
High GI > 70

Glycemic "load" uses the glycemic index to go a step further, taking into account the amount of carbohydrates that a food contains in a typical serving. Comparing foods, we find that those with a low glycemic index will also have a low glycemic load, but foods with a high glycemic index may have either a high glycemic load or a low glycemic load, once the available carbohydrate content is considered. The available carbohydrate content means the usable carbohydrates that are left once the fiber has been removed; the equation for determining the glycemic load includes the carbohydrate content. Fortunately, many lists are available that provide the glycemic index and load of a specific food, so you don't have to do all that math!

Foods that have rapidly digestible sugar but also a high water content will have a high glycemic index value but a low glycemic load, because there is relatively little sugar in an average serving of the food. Fat also plays a role in how quickly a food is digested, but this is not incorporated in the basic glycemic load equation. Let's run the conversion from glycemic index to glycemic load using watermelon as an example.

The general conversion equation is

$$\text{glycemic load of a food} = \frac{\begin{pmatrix} \text{glycemic index of that food} \times \text{grams} \\ \text{of available carbohydrates it contains} \end{pmatrix}}{100}$$

The different levels of glycemic load are classified as low, medium, and high. These classifications reflect how quickly and by how much a particular food will elevate your blood sugar. The ranges of the levels of glycemic load (GL) are shown here:

Low GL < 10
Moderate GL < 11–19
High GL > 20

So, for 120 grams (roughly 4 ounces) of watermelon

The glycemic index of 120 grams of watermelon is 72.

The amount of available carbohydrates in this much watermelon is 6 grams.

Therefore, the glycemic load of 120 grams of watermelon is

$$\text{glycemic load} = \frac{(72 \times 6)}{100} = 4.32$$

This means that watermelon will not raise your blood sugar levels too high or too quickly. Low glycemic load foods tend to keep blood sugar levels on an even keel, without any huge spikes. This is beneficial because then your body does not have to produce a lot of insulin to deal with the excess sugar. It is therefore less likely that your cells will become resistant to insulin, and your risk of developing type 2 diabetes is lower.

An example of glycemic index/glycemic load tables can be found at the Harvard Health website: https://www.health.harvard.edu/diseases -and-conditions/glycemic-index-and-glycemic-load-for-100-foods.

For a list of the GI/GL values of approximately one thousand foods, including brand name items, see the open access article published in *Diabetes Care*, the journal of the American Diabetes Association.[1] You can download the complete table, free of charge, at https://www.ncbi .nlm.nih.gov/pmc/articles/PMC2584181/.

As with all dietary changes, common sense should prevail. This information is presented for you to think about what you are eating and how it affects your body. It is not meant to endorse low glycemic load diets as the only way to eat.

---

1. F. A. Atkinson, K. Foster-Powell, and J. C. Brand-Miller, "International Tables of Glycemic Index and Glycemic Load Values: 2008," *Diabetes Care* 31(12): 2281–2283, doi:10.3227/dc08-1239.

Glycemic Index

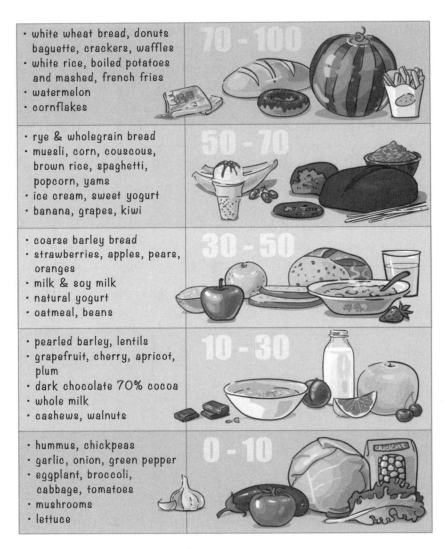

- white wheat bread, donuts baguette, crackers, waffles
- white rice, boiled potatoes and mashed, french fries
- watermelon
- cornflakes

70 - 100

- rye & wholegrain bread
- muesli, corn, couscous, brown rice, spaghetti, popcorn, yams
- ice cream, sweet yogurt
- banana, grapes, kiwi

50 - 70

- coarse barley bread
- strawberries, apples, pears, oranges
- milk & soy milk
- natural yogurt
- oatmeal, beans

30 - 50

- pearled barley, lentils
- grapefruit, cherry, apricot, plum
- dark chocolate 70% cocoa
- whole milk
- cashews, walnuts

10 - 30

- hummus, chickpeas
- garlic, onion, green pepper
- eggplant, broccoli, cabbage, tomatoes
- mushrooms
- lettuce

0 - 10

Illustration courtesy of Shutterstock

True Wellness Checklist

Instructions for Use

The True Wellness Checklist is a compilation of recommended actions that are associated with optimal health. These actions form the basis of disease prevention in both Eastern and Western medical systems. Meditation, qigong, cardiovascular exercise, and resistance training should be incorporated into everyone's healing plan. Although sleep is not on the checklist, you should strive for seven to eight hours of sleep within a twenty-four-hour period.

Many people have food sensitivities, allergies, or individual preferences; therefore, the dietary recommendations on the checklist form the essentials of a vegan regimen. You can add servings of meat, fish, or dairy, depending on your tastes or requirements. The majority of your food should be plant-based. If you do eat animal products, your plate should be filled three-quarters with plants and only one-quarter with animal protein. Choose whole foods over processed foods. Minimize sweets, but enjoy chocolate made of at least 70 percent cacao on occasion.

Approximate serving sizes:

Vegetables	1 cup raw vegetables, ½ cup cooked vegetables
Fruit	1 medium piece of raw fruit, ½ cup canned fruit, ¼ cup dried fruit
Nuts	1/3 cup
Beans/Legumes	½ cup cooked

Whole Grains	1 slice of bread, ½ cup cooked grains, 1 ounce dry cereal
Red meat, poultry	cooked, roughly the same size as a deck of cards
Fish	uncooked, 8 ounces (no more than 3x/week because of heavy metals)
Dairy	1 cup of yogurt, 1 cup of milk, 2 ounces of cheese
Eggs	1 egg
Oils	extra virgin olive oil, flaxseed oil for cooking and dressings

TRUE WELLNESS CHECKLIST

	SUNDAY	MONDAY	TUESDAY	WEDNESDAY	THURSDAY	FRIDAY	SATURDAY
MEDITATE daily	○	○	○	○	○	○	○
QIGONG TAI CHI 3-7x/week	○	○	○	○	○	○	○
CARDIO/ RESISTANCE TRAINING 3-5x/week	○	○	○	○	○	○	○
VEGETABLES 4-6 servings daily	○○○○○○	○○○○○○	○○○○	○○○○○○	○○○○○○	○○○○○○	○○○○○○
FRUIT 3-4 servings daily	○○○○	○○○○	○○○○	○○○○	○○○○	○○○○	○○○○
NUTS 1/3 cup daily	○	○	○	○	○	○	○
BEANS/LEGUMES 1-2 servings daily	○○	○○	○○	○○	○○	○○	○○
WHOLE GRAINS 3-4 servings daily	○○○○	○○○○	○○○○	○○○○	○○○○	○○○○	○○○○
WATER 8 oz. glass 8 servings daily	○○○○○○○○	○○○○○○○○	○○○○○○○○	○○○○○○○○	○○○○○○○○	○○○○○○○○	○○○○○○○○

Glossary

Accreditation Commission for Acupuncture and Oriental Medicine (ACAOM). National agency, recognized by the United States Department of Education (USDE), that accredits master's-level programs in acupuncture and Oriental medicine, ensuring that such programs meet the standards for education set by Congress.

acupuncture. System of medicine that involves inserting fine metal needles into specific anatomic locations to treat a variety of illnesses and conditions. Derived from the Latin *acus* (needle) + puncture.

American Academy of Medical Acupuncture (AAMA). Society of medical doctors (MDs) and osteopaths (DOs) who have undergone training in acupuncture to incorporate this modality into conventional health care. Founded in 1987.

American Board of Medical Acupuncturists (ABMA). Independent entity within the AAMA. Established in 2000 to conduct examinations of candidates seeking certification in medical acupuncture, to maintain high standards for the profession.

American Medical Association (AMA). Professional association of medical doctors (MDs) and osteopaths (DOs) founded in 1847. The stated mission of the AMA is to "promote the art and science of medicine and the betterment of public health."

Ben Cao Gang Mu (*Compendium of Materia Medica*). Encyclopedic medical volume detailing the herbs and other substances used in Chinese medicine. Written in the sixteenth century CE by Li Shi-Zhen, a prominent physician in the Ming dynasty.

Buddhism. Religion that developed out of the teachings of Siddhartha Gautama in the fifth century BCE, spreading from northeastern India through Asia and globally. Gautama became known as Buddha and taught that life is full of suffering, but suffering can be overcome by developing wisdom, integrity, and awareness.

chromosomes. Coiled structures within the nucleus of most cells that contain the genetic information required for life.

Confucianism. Teachings of Confucius, emphasizing correct behavior of the institutions and individuals within society, as well as the cultivation of knowledge and good judgment.

Confucius. Chinese philosopher, political figure, and educator who lived during the fifth and sixth centuries BCE. His teachings are known as Confucianism.

Dao De Ching. (Also known as *Tao Te Ching.*) Chinese text regarding the philosophy of Daoism, attributed to Laozi (see Daoism). May actually be a compilation of works by later authors.

Daoism. (Also known as Taoism.) Doctrine of living in harmony with the natural order of the universe. Ascribed to the teachings of Laozi, a Chinese philosopher who lived during the sixth century BCE.

DNA (deoxyribonucleic acid). Long double-stranded and twisted chain of organic molecules that make up chromosomes. The sequence of the organic molecules acts as a blueprint for the body to create other necessary substances such as proteins and enzymes.

Eastern medicine. System of medicine that arose in Asia that makes use of herbal remedies, acupuncture, meditation, qigong, and tai chi to improve health. Also known as Oriental medicine, East Asian medicine.

Five Phases. The cosmological scheme that describes interactions among natural phenomena, such as the changing of the seasons. Developed in ancient China millennia ago and used in astrology, military strategy, and medicine. Also referred to as "five elements."

Food and Drug Administration (FDA). Agency of the US Department of Health and Human Services created to ensure that food, drugs, and medical devices are safe and effective. Also assures that cosmetic and dietary supplements are safe and labeled properly, protects the public from electronic product radiation, and regulates tobacco products.

functional magnetic resonance imaging (fMRI). An imaging technique that employs magnetic and radio waves. Used to determine which areas of the brain are most active at the time of the study.

gene. A sequence of DNA that codes for a molecule that has a specific function within a living organism (see DNA).

Huang Di Nei Jing (The Yellow Emperor's Classic of Internal Medicine). Ancient Chinese medical text written approximately during the Han dynasty (206 BCE–220 CE).

Hua Tuo. Famed second-century CE Chinese physician and surgeon who also developed longevity exercises called Five Animal qigong.

integrative medicine. A branch of conventional Western medicine that is patient-centered and incorporates techniques from other medical systems for which there is good evidence of safety and efficacy.

Journal of the American Medical Association (JAMA). Peer-reviewed medical journal published by the AMA containing research papers, reviews, and editorials that relate to the field of medicine.

Laozi. See Daoism.

licensed acupuncturist (LAc). Designation given to a person who has received a license to practice acupuncture from a state medical or professional licensing board. To qualify, that person must have completed a specific amount of training and passed certifying examinations in acupuncture and Oriental medicine.

mind-body medicine. Group of therapeutic practices that engage the mind's capacity to influence bodily functions. Examples of these techniques include meditation, relaxation, biofeedback, and hypnosis.

National Certification Commission for Acupuncture and Oriental Medicine (NCCAOM). Nonprofit organization established in 1982 to certify competency of acupuncturists, herbologists, and bodyworkers of Eastern medical disciplines in the United States. The NCCAOM is also involved with recertification, examination development, and continuing education.

neuroplasticity. Ability of the brain to form new connections and pathways in response to learning or training. Also known as brain plasticity.

Oriental medicine. System of medicine that arose in Asia (the Orient) that makes use of herbal remedies, acupuncture, meditation, qigong, and tai chi to improve health. Also known as Eastern medicine, East Asian medicine.

placebo. A substance or intervention that has no active ingredient or expected benefit.

placebo effect. Positive, unexpected benefit seen following administration of a placebo. Attributed to the recipient's expectation of benefit, considered a mind-body interaction.

post-heaven qi. Eastern medicine term for energy (qi) extracted by the body from food and air.

pre-heaven qi. Eastern medicine term for energy (qi) that is inherited from our parents. Analogous to genetic constitution in Western medicine.

preventive medicine. Medical specialty that focuses on the prevention of disease, not only in the individual patient but in the community and population at large. A combination of clinical medicine and public health.

PubMed. Free search engine that can be used to find abstracts and articles on life sciences and biomedical subjects. Maintained by the National Center for Biotechnology Information at the US National Library of Medicine.

qi. Eastern medicine term for the intelligent life force that flows through the body. Often described in Western terms as "energy."

qigong. Mental, physical, and breathing exercises that cultivate qi. Related to tai chi (see tai chi).

Silk Road. Ancient trading route between Asia and Europe that traversed Korea, China, India, Persia, and Europe.

Sun Si-Miao. Prolific seventh-century CE Chinese physician and herbalist who wrote two thirty-volume works on the practice of medicine. Renowned for integrating Daoism with Buddhism and Confucianism. Emphasized ethical behavior for physicians.

tai chi. (Also spelled *taiji*.) Chinese martial art form, but also a series of slow, meditative movements that, when performed regularly, can improve health and well-being. Related to qigong (see qigong).

telomerase. Enzyme that adds specific molecules to the ends of telomeres to preserve their length (see telomere).

telomere. Noncoding DNA sequence on the ends of chromosomes that protect the chromosome and protect the loss of genetic information during DNA transcription.

tui na. Method of Chinese bodywork or massage.

World Health Organization (WHO). Agency of the United Nations, established in 1948, intended to improve international public health.

Wu Xing. See Five Phases.

yin-yang theory. Theory that states that all phenomena are composed of two opposite conditions or characteristics. These opposites cannot be separated. Together, they represent the unified whole.

Recommended Reading and Resources

Abramson, John. *Overdosed America: The Broken Promise of American Medicine.* New York: Harper Collins, 2004.

Beck, Martha. *The Four-Day Win: End Your Diet War and Achieve Thinner Peace.* New York: Rodale, 2007.

Blackburn, Elizabeth, and Elissa Epel. *The Telomere Effect: A Revolutionary Approach to Living Younger, Healthier, Longer.* New York: Grand Central Publishing, 2017.

Doidge, Norman. *The Brain That Changes Itself.* New York: Viking/Penguin, 2007.

Doidge, Norman. *The Brain's Way of Healing.* New York: Penguin, 2015.

Gawande, Atul. *Complications: A Surgeon's Notes on an Imperfect Science,* New York: Henry Holt, 2002.

Harris, Dan. *10% Happier: How I Tamed the Voice in My Head, Reduced Stress Without Losing My Edge, and Found Self-Help That Actually Works—A True Story.* New York: HarperCollins, 2014.

Helms, Joseph. *Getting to Know You: A Physician Explains How Acupuncture Helps You Be the Best You.* Berkeley, CA: M.A.P. Medical Acupuncture Publishers, 2007.

Kaptchuk, Ted. *The Web That Has No Weaver: Understanding Chinese Medicine.* New York: McGraw-Hill, 2000.

Keown, Daniel. *The Spark in the Machine: How the Science of Acupuncture Explains the Mysteries of Western Medicine.* London: Singing Dragon, 2014.

Kuhn, Aihan. *Brain Fitness: The Easy Way of Keeping Your Mind Sharp through Qigong.* Wolfeboro, NH: YMAA Publication Center, 2017.

Kuhn, Aihan. *Natural Healing with Qigong: Therapeutic Qigong.* Wolfeboro, NH: YMAA Publication Center, 2004.

Kuhn, Aihan. *Simple Chinese Medicine: A Beginner's Guide to Natural Healing and Well-Being.* Wolfeboro, NH: YMAA Publication Center, 2009.

Kuhn, Aihan. *Tai Chi for Depression: A 10-Week Program to Empower Yourself and Beat Depression.* Wolfeboro, NH: YMAA Publication Center, 2017.

Kuhn, Aihan. *Tai Chi in 10 Weeks: Beginner's Guide, A Proven Step-by-Step Plan for Integrating the Physical and Psychological Benefits of Tai Chi into Your Life.* Wolfeboro, NH: YMAA Publication Center, 2017.

Lee, Jennie. *Breathing Love: Meditation in Action.* Woodbury, MN: Llewellyn World-wide, 2018.

Reid, T. R. *The Healing of America: A Global Quest for Better, Cheaper, and Fairer Health Care.* London: Penguin, 2010.

Scheid, Volker, and Hugh MacPherson, editors. *Integrating East Asian Medicine into Contemporary Health Care.* Edinburgh: Churchill Livingston/Elsevier, 2012.

Weil, Andrew. *You Can't Afford to Get Sick: Your Guide to Optimum Health and Health Care.* New York: Plume, 2009.

Index

About the Authors

Dr. Catherine Kurosu

Born, raised, and trained in Canada, Dr. Catherine Kurosu graduated from the University of Toronto School of Medicine in 1990. She completed her internship and residency at the same institution and qualified as a specialist in obstetrics and gynecology in 1995. Dr. Kurosu has studied and worked in Canada, the United States, Mexico, and Chile.

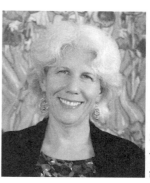

Photo by: Monica Lau

Through her travels, she has learned that there are many ways to approach a problem and that the patient usually understands their illness best. By combining the patient's insight with medical guidance, effective treatment plans can be developed.

In 2006, Dr. Kurosu became a diplomate of the American Board of Holistic Medicine, now known as the American Board of Integrative Holistic Medicine. In 2009, she became certified as a medical acupuncturist through the David Geffen School of Medicine at UCLA and the Helms Medical Institute. Dr. Kurosu became a member of the American Academy of Medical Acupuncture, then a diplomate of the American Board of Medical Acupuncture, which confers this title to practitioners with increasing experience.

Since then, Dr. Kurosu completed a master of science in Oriental medicine, graduating from the Institute of Clinical Acupuncture and Oriental Medicine in Honolulu. In 2015, she became a licensed acupuncturist in Hawai'i, where she practices integrative medicine, blending Western and Eastern approaches to patient care.

She now lives on O'ahu with husband, Rob, and daughter, Hannah.

Dr. Aihan Kuhn

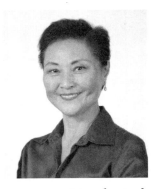

A graduate of Hunan Medical University in China (now called Xiangya Medical School) in 1982, Dr. Aihan Kuhn had oriented her focus to holistic healing since 1992. During many years of practice, she has accumulated much experience with holistic medicine and achieved a great reputation for her patient care and education work. Her patients benefit from her many important tips for self-improvement in physical, emotional, and spiritual well-being, as well as simple and easy healing exercises to enable them to participate in healing. Dr. Kuhn incorporates tai chi and qigong into her healing methodologies, changing the lives of those who have struggled for many years with no relief from conventional medicine. Dr. Kuhn provides many wellness programs, natural healing workshops, and professional training programs, such as tai chi instructor training certification courses, qigong instructor training certification courses, and wellness tui na therapy certification courses. These highly rated programs have produced many quality teachers and therapists. Dr. Kuhn is president of the Tai Chi & Qi Gong Healing Institute (www.TaiChiHealing.org), a nonprofit organization that promotes natural healing and prevention.

Dr. Kuhn lives with her husband, Gerry, in Sarasota, Florida. For more information, visit www.draihankuhn.com.

BOOKS FROM YMAA

6 HEALING MOVEMENTS
101 REFLECTIONS ON TAI CHI CHUAN
108 INSIGHTS INTO TAI CHI CHUAN
ADVANCING IN TAE KWON DO
ANALYSIS OF SHAOLIN CHIN NA 2ND ED
ANCIENT CHINESE WEAPONS
THE ART AND SCIENCE OF STAFF FIGHTING
ART OF HOJO UNDO
ARTHRITIS RELIEF, 3D ED.
BACK PAIN RELIEF, 2ND ED.
BAGUAZHANG, 2ND ED.
BRAIN FITNESS
CARDIO KICKBOXING ELITE
CHIN NA IN GROUND FIGHTING
CHINESE FAST WRESTLING
CHINESE FITNESS
CHINESE TUI NA MASSAGE
CHOJUN
COMPREHENSIVE APPLICATIONS OF SHAOLIN CHIN NA
CONFLICT COMMUNICATION
CROCODILE AND THE CRANE: A NOVEL
CUTTING SEASON: A XENON PEARL MARTIAL ARTS THRILLER
DAO DE JING
DEFENSIVE TACTICS
DESHI: A CONNOR BURKE MARTIAL ARTS THRILLER
DIRTY GROUND
DR. WU'S HEAD MASSAGE
DUKKHA HUNGRY GHOSTS
DUKKHA REVERB
DUKKHA, THE SUFFERING: AN EYE FOR AN EYE
DUKKHA UNLOADED
ENZAN: THE FAR MOUNTAIN, A CONNOR BURKE MARTIAL ARTS
    THRILLER
ESSENCE OF SHAOLIN WHITE CRANE
EVEN IF IT KILLS ME
EXPLORING TAI CHI
FACING VIOLENCE
FIGHT BACK
FIGHT LIKE A PHYSICIST
THE FIGHTER'S BODY
FIGHTER'S FACT BOOK
FIGHTER'S FACT BOOK 2
FIGHTING THE PAIN RESISTANT ATTACKER
FIRST DEFENSE
FORCE DECISIONS: A CITIZENS GUIDE
FOX BORROWS THE TIGER'S AWE
INSIDE TAI CHI
KAGE: THE SHADOW, A CONNOR BURKE MARTIAL ARTS
    THRILLER
KARATE SCIENCE
KATA AND THE TRANSMISSION OF KNOWLEDGE
KRAV MAGA PROFESSIONAL TACTICS
KRAV MAGA WEAPON DEFENSES
LITTLE BLACK BOOK OF VIOLENCE
LIUHEBAFA FIVE CHARACTER SECRETS
MARTIAL ARTS ATHLETE
MARTIAL ARTS INSTRUCTION
MARTIAL WAY AND ITS VIRTUES
MASK OF THE KING
MEDITATIONS ON VIOLENCE
MERIDIAN QIGONG EXERCISES
MIND/BODY FITNESS
MINDFUL EXERCISE
THE MIND INSIDE TAI CHI
THE MIND INSIDE YANG STYLE TAI CHI CHUAN
MUGAI RYU
NATURAL HEALING WITH QIGONG
NORTHERN SHAOLIN SWORD, 2ND ED.
OKINAWA'S COMPLETE KARATE SYSTEM: ISSHIN RYU
THE PAIN-FREE BACK
PAIN-FREE JOINTS
POWER BODY
PRINCIPLES OF TRADITIONAL CHINESE MEDICINE

THE PROTECTOR ETHIC
QIGONG FOR HEALTH & MARTIAL ARTS 2ND ED.
QIGONG FOR LIVING
QIGONG FOR TREATING COMMON AILMENTS
QIGONG MASSAGE
QIGONG MEDITATION: EMBRYONIC BREATHING
QIGONG MEDITATION: SMALL CIRCULATION
QIGONG, THE SECRET OF YOUTH: DA MO'S CLASSICS
QUIET TEACHER: A XENON PEARL MARTIAL ARTS THRILLER
RAVEN'S WARRIOR
REDEMPTION
ROOT OF CHINESE QIGONG, 2ND ED.
SCALING FORCE
SENSEI: A CONNOR BURKE MARTIAL ARTS THRILLER
SHIHAN TE: THE BUNKAI OF KATA
SHIN GI TAI: KARATE TRAINING FOR BODY, MIND, AND SPIRIT
SIMPLE CHINESE MEDICINE
SIMPLE QIGONG EXERCISES FOR HEALTH, 3RD ED.
SIMPLIFIED TAI CHI CHUAN, 2ND ED.
SIMPLIFIED TAI CHI FOR BEGINNERS
SOLO TRAINING
SOLO TRAINING 2
SUDDEN DAWN: THE EPIC JOURNEY OF BODHIDHARMA
SUMO FOR MIXED MARTIAL ARTS
SUNRISE TAI CHI
SUNSET TAI CHI
SURVIVING ARMED ASSAULTS
TAE KWON DO: THE KOREAN MARTIAL ART
TAEKWONDO BLACK BELT POOMSAE
TAEKWONDO: A PATH TO EXCELLENCE
TAEKWONDO: ANCIENT WISDOM FOR THE MODERN WARRIOR
TAEKWONDO: DEFENSES AGAINST WEAPONS
TAEKWONDO: SPIRIT AND PRACTICE
TAO OF BIOENERGETICS
TAI CHI BALL QIGONG: FOR HEALTH AND MARTIAL ARTS
TAI CHI BALL WORKOUT FOR BEGINNERS
TAI CHI BOOK
TAI CHI CHIN NA: THE SEIZING ART OF TAI CHI CHUAN,
    2ND ED.
TAI CHI CHUAN CLASSICAL YANG STYLE, 2ND ED.
TAI CHI CHUAN MARTIAL APPLICATIONS
TAI CHI CHUAN MARTIAL POWER, 3RD ED.
TAI CHI CONNECTIONS
TAI CHI DYNAMICS
TAI CHI FOR DEPRESSION
TAI CHI IN 10 WEEKS
TAI CHI QIGONG, 3RD ED.
TAI CHI SECRETS OF THE ANCIENT MASTERS
TAI CHI SECRETS OF THE WU & LI STYLES
TAI CHI SECRETS OF THE WU STYLE
TAI CHI SECRETS OF THE YANG STYLE
TAI CHI SWORD: CLASSICAL YANG STYLE, 2ND ED.
TAI CHI SWORD FOR BEGINNERS
TAI CHI WALKING
TAIJIQUAN THEORY OF DR. YANG, JWING-MING
TENGU: THE MOUNTAIN GOBLIN, A CONNOR BURKE MARTIAL
    ARTS THRILLER
TIMING IN THE FIGHTING ARTS
TRADITIONAL CHINESE HEALTH SECRETS
TRADITIONAL TAEKWONDO
TRAINING FOR SUDDEN VIOLENCE
TRUE WELLNESS
THE WARRIOR'S MANIFESTO
WAY OF KATA
WAY OF KENDO AND KENJITSU
WAY OF SANCHIN KATA
WAY TO BLACK BELT
WESTERN HERBS FOR MARTIAL ARTISTS
WILD GOOSE QIGONG
WINNING FIGHTS
WOMAN'S QIGONG GUIDE
XINGYIQUAN

DVDS FROM YMAA

more products available from . . .
YMAA Publication Center, Inc. 楊氏東方文化出版中心
1-800-669-8892 • info@ymaa.com • www.ymaa.com